I'M GONNA BE A FIRST-TIME DAD

THE EXPECTANT FATHER'S GUIDE TO 9 MONTHS OF PREGNANCY, BIRTH & BEYOND. HOW TO PREPARE FOR FATHERHOOD WITH COMPLETE CONFIDENCE

NIGEL BOYD

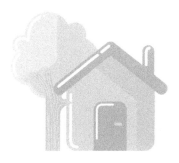

My dad. You paved the way for me to be the best dad possible by your example.

To my wife Leah. For making this book possible, I love you and our children.

CONTENTS

INTRODUCTION

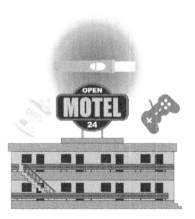

It's hard to think of a six-word sentence more powerful than "You're going to be a dad."

Joy, fear, euphoria, panic; an immediate roller coaster of emotions follows those words, and it can be a lot to process. For me, that roller coaster came with a wave of questions. What can I do to help my wife during pregnancy? What appointments do we need to make? Are my finances in order? And the one that scared me the most…am I ready to be a dad?

THOSE SIX LITTLE WORDS

I first heard those words in 2011, sitting on the bed in a hotel room just outside Las Vegas. At the time, I was a long-haul truck driver; my co-driver and I were staying in Nevada on a layover. We had just finished back to back trips to L.A., and we were finally headed back home to Wisconsin. There I was, 24 years old, blissfully gaming and eating handfuls of junk food, not a care in the world. At the time, I really did think I had everything figured out. Who doesn't at 24?

Then my phone rang. It was my wife, Leah.

I started the conversation totally oblivious, bragging about beating a level we had both been stuck on, but Leah cut me off. I'll never forget how excited she sounded. Her voice was a couple of octaves higher than usual, and completely breathless. She didn't waste any time, telling me that the first test was positive, and the second test, and the third.

"You're going to be a dad."

After the call was over, I remember the phone was still gripped in my hand for several minutes, and I couldn't stop smiling. I was in a state of shock, mixed with absolute elation. Sleep was the furthest thing from my mind as my thoughts moved a mile a minute. I was thrilled, but honestly, I was also worried.

Don't get me wrong, I've always wanted to be a father; My parents had ten kids, I was their sixth. That wouldn't work for some people, but my parents couldn't have been happier. They worked hard and made sure we had everything we needed. To this day, I know I can call my parents day or night and they'll do everything they can to help me out.

Still, us kids had to pitch in from time to time. Naturally, we had more than our fair share of arguments. But I learned a lot of good skills taking care of my younger siblings, not to mention the invaluable advice I got from my older brothers and sisters. Our family is incredibly close, and it's a constant comfort to know I have a big group of people I can always depend on. I just can't imagine life any other way.

What I'm trying to say is, having a big family of my own was always the plan. But a plan is one thing, and hearing those six words is something else entirely. So when I got that call, part of me was over the moon; I could already see our little son or daughter playing in the yard, learning to ride a bike, heading off to their first day of school. There was a wealth of memories to be made, and I couldn't wait to make them.

But at the same time, I felt a world of responsibility wash over me. Life was never going to be the same, and here I was playing video games and wiping cheeto dust onto my pants. It was tough to admit, but at the time, I thought I wasn't ready to be a dad.

SO WHAT DID I DO?

The same thing you're doing: I began learning as much as I could, as quickly as possible. I started that night, frantically searching on a computer in the hotel's lobby; hopefully, you are getting ready a bit sooner than I did.

I kept researching through the first pregnancy, encountering new problems, finding solutions, and writing down what I'd found. I always loved research papers in school, and once I get focused on a subject, it's tough to tear me away. I didn't realize it at the time, but I was planting the seeds that would grow into this very book.

Some of the notes I took that first night made their way into these chapters. The rest comes from pieces of scrap paper, spiral notebooks filled with my terrible handwriting, whatever I could type out in my phone, and endless documents on my computer. Even after our first son Alan was born, I didn't stop. It became my mission to learn as much as possible, and document what I had learned. My hope is that all that research, and the book that came from it, makes your journey a bit easier. By the end, you'll know everything I know about being a better partner, and a better father.

WHERE DO YOU BEGIN?

The most crucial first step is to realize that *this really isn't about you*. Let me be 100% clear: being a father is incredibly important. But it also involves putting others above yourself. Right now, your job is to be the best partner you can possibly be. In the coming months, you'll need to support your wife or girlfriend through some of the most challenging experiences in human existence: pregnancy, childbirth, and if the worst should happen, miscarriage.

By contributing as much time and effort as possible, you will not only help your partner but the life that's growing inside of them. Stress can be a dangerous cocktail for both a mother and a child. Studies have shown that prenatal stress can cause a premature or underweight baby, along with a host of other complications. So reducing that stress will be one of your main goals for the next 9 months.

Your support role will include a variety of duties, like:

- Helping with doctor's appointments
- Understanding medical terminology related to pregnancy
- Assisting with various ailments associated with pregnancy
- Tracking certain health metrics for both her and the baby
- Keeping her morale up
- Helping her get enough nourishment

And countless more steps we'll cover to ensure you are doing your part. But that's not the end of your responsibilities either. You also need to prepare yourself and your home for the arrival of a child. Little feet will soon be pitter-pattering under your roof, and you need to make sure everything is 100% ready before you come home from the hospital. That means looking at yourself, in and out, and making sure you are prepared for your life to change forever.

IT'S OKAY TO FEEL OVERWHELMED. I WAS AT FIRST.

I know this sounds like a lot. But, believe me, so many good times lay ahead. The pregnancy itself has countless unforgettable, life-altering moments: Seeing your child on an ultrasound for the first time, learning whether they'll be a boy or a girl, telling loved ones the news.

Or even that first moment, wherever it ends up happening. Whether you are looking your wife right in the eyes, you hear an excited yell from the other room, or you get a call while sitting in a hotel in Nevada. This all begins with those six little words.

You're going to be a dad.

SO YOU'RE GOING TO BE A DAD! NOW WHAT?

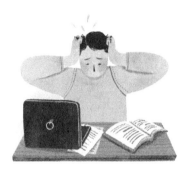

A lot of emotions will hit you right after finding out you're going to be a dad. Joy and fear will take turns in the driver's seat; until you begin to really understand what tasks lie ahead, you'll probably have a decent amount of anxiety. I personally switched between baby books and binge-watching old episodes of The Office to decompress. But that's actually an essential part of this process:

FIND LITTLE PIECES OF TIME TO RELAX

Yes, life will get more hectic soon, but you don't want to approach this in a panic. Stress inhibits our ability to learn and store new information. It may not feel like it, but you do have time. You want to make sure to think carefully about what questions you have, and find satisfying answers for each. The best way to do this is to listen to former first-time dads, and what their experience was.

Anytime we embark on a new journey, it's natural to seek out the wisdom of those who have been there before us. So what fears do other first-time dads have? I looked online, asked a couple of family and friends, and thought about my initial worries the first time. Here are a couple of the most common questions I could find. For many of these, there is no easy answer. But I have done my best to quell some of these worries, so you can focus on what you need to do next.

4 COMMON FEARS FOR FIRST-TIME DADS

Fear #1: How is my kid going to turn out in the future?

This is a perfectly normal concern to have. What will your child be like when they grow up? Every dad has an idea of who their child might be, but for most, you want them to grow up to be:

- A good person; someone who has strong morals
- Successful, so they can eventually find independence
- Happy. Every parent wants their child to find happiness in life

But, the fact of the matter is, you can't know how your kid is going to grow up. That future adult, the one your child ends up growing into, depends on a wide variety of factors. The main ones that you can control are the environment you provide for them and the experiences you facilitate. It's about putting in the time and effort with each step in your child's growth, and once they get to a certain age, you can show them the right path. If you do your absolute best, you get an incredible reward: the confidence that you have done everything in your power to guide them towards a good life.

Even after they have grown up and left the nest, you can provide advice and assistance whenever possible to help them find further success. But there's another lesson to take in here:

Don't hit fast forward

Thinking about the future is good, and can help you prepare for the obstacles you will face as a parent. But focusing on the present is absolutely essential. It's a cliche, but the phrase will always ring true: Life is short. Don't miss those little moments because you are thinking about 10, 20, or 30 years into the future. Live for the now, and embrace every precious second you have with your children.

Fear #2: How can I raise my kid right?

Again, this depends heavily on your particular beliefs. You most likely have an idea of how you want to raise your child, and this idea will be guided by your specific set of values. These values may be based on how you were raised, or ones you have designed yourself as an adult. You can also supplement these guidelines with the things you learn from others. Whatever the case is, you will be learning and growing with your kid, and your child-rearing technique will evolve over time. You'll take in more information and get advice from parents you know and trust. I remember calling my dad every couple of days during our first pregnancy to annoy him, pen and paper ready with questions rapid firing from my worried brain. I'm thankful that no matter what he was doing, he would take the time to give me advice. That's my benchmark for how I raise my children: being there any time they need me, no matter what.

But even with all the advice in the world, I can promise you one thing that is inevitable. When it comes to raising kids, there is simply no way to avoid it:

You will make mistakes

Mistakes are going to happen. Every parent makes mistakes, including me. You'll say the wrong thing, get frustrated, and yes-feel a painful sense of regret. But don't let a simple stumble destroy your confidence as a father. Messing up is part of life. There is this ancient Japanese art you may have heard of, called Kintsugi. In it, breaking a pot isn't seen as a negative.

Kintsugi (金継ぎ , "golden joinery"), also known as kintsukuroi (金繕い, "golden repair"), is the Japanese art of repairing broken pottery by mending the areas of breakage with lacquer dusted or mixed with powdered gold, silver, or platinum; the method is similar to the maki-e technique a pot breaks, they don't throw it away.

Instead, they fix it with gold, and the new pot is often even better than before. Of course, mistakes will happen; the important part is *learning* from them and doing what you can to be *better* in the future.

Fear #3: Will I be able to support my family financially, physically, and emotionally?

This, thankfully, you have a lot more control over. Once you know you are having a child, it's time to take stock. Sit down and make an assessment of your financial, physical, and emotional condition right now. What status are each of these facets in your life at? Let's look at some specific questions that you can ask yourself for each of these situations:

Financial

Your financial stability hinges on a couple of factors:

- Do you have a steady, secure job?
- Do you have an investment strategy?
- Do you have an emergency fund?
- Do you have a structured budget?

You want to make sure that you are in a position of employment where enough money is coming in to cover your expenses, and then some. This may involve a degree of compromise. If you are working a job you like but aren't making near enough money to support a family, you may have some soul searching to do. Driving a truck wasn't exactly my dream as a kid, and I had been thinking of getting into a different line of work before our first child. It wasn't ideal, but I stayed with my career, and I'm glad I did. For my own happiness, I made some changes to my work. I found a company that would let me do day-trips as opposed to long-haul treks across the country, which let me come home every day to my family. Even after switching to shorter runs, I still make more than enough to support them. But, that doesn't mean I can be reckless with my money.

Establishing a budget is an excellent first step to understanding the flow of your finances. Before I budgeted, I would often think: Where does it all go? I didn't realize that it's pretty easy to see where it goes; you just have to be looking. I took a long hard look at my income and expenses and started to see just how much money I was wasting. Going out to eat, both on the road and at home, was easily my biggest vice. I love a good restaurant, whether alone or with Leah. The atmosphere, the service, expertly cooked meals and no dishes at the end. It really lets you enjoy your meal, and it was a pleasure we admittedly overindulged in. Once I began to assess my credit card statement, I could see that my foodie habit was poking a massive hole in my savings. So I started changing my patterns, starting with Leah shopping and meal-prepping more often. Including this, she limited her daily coffee runs to Starbucks. We were amazed at the thousands of dollars that appeared in our bank account. Of course, we still eat out from time to time or have our specialty caffeine kicks. But it's a treat, not a routine, and I think that's the important distinction to make.

When looking at your savings account, there is an easy metric you can use to see if you have enough in the case of an emergency. For an emergency fund to provide substantial relief, you'll want to make sure you have the money to cover your expenses for 6 months to a year. This fund can be a lifesaver in several cases, including:

- Sudden medical expense
- A death occurs in the family (funeral costs, etc)
- Your vehicle requires major repairs
- Unexpected but essential travel
- Something happens with your work (job loss, pay cut, etc)
- Surprise home repairs

Once your emergency fund and savings are in order, you want to make sure you have a sound investment strategy. The best course of action is to talk to a professional financial advisor, but that isn't always readily available. If you do want to invest on your own, carefully research some safe, total market ETFs (exchange-traded funds) that can slowly grow your money. Stay away from picking individual stocks; that's basically gambling.

After every one of these pieces of the puzzle falls into place, then you can look at making discretionary purchases. And by all means, do so! That's the great part of having your life together; once you are comfortable knowing everything is secure, you can spend money on those silly items that make life a little sweeter. I, for example, collect Nintendo systems and games. I have several shelves built in the living room to display my collection (alongside Leah's impressive collection of Disney memorabilia.) Whatever your hobby or pastime is, make sure to spend some of your hard-earned money expanding your interests. One day, you may even get to see your child joyfully participate in that hobby you love so much!

Physical

Your physical health plays a large part in your ability to be a father. You want to show your child healthy habits and be able to play with them as they grow. Being healthy also means you can make sure you'll be around as long as possible. Losing a parent is a harrowing experience, and the longer you can delay that, the better off your child will be. You want to be there to help and guide them through the difficulties of life, and the only way to guarantee that is by staying healthy.

If you have any vices, take a good long look at their effect on your life. Two common vices we see everywhere are cigarettes and alcohol. 20% of all deaths in the United States are from smoking, one every 4.5 seconds. While these statistics might not mean much to you now, there are more immediate detriments to these behaviors. I've had friends who smoked, so I understand. But when their kids came along, they knew they had to get off the nicotine.

A good friend of mine recommends Allen Carr's *Easy Way to Stop Smoking*, which he says really helped him quit. He said it gave him perspective on his habit and to understand why he had fallen into addiction in the first place. If you do decide to keep smoking, I understand. Life is stressful, and quitting adds more stress on top. But, smoking may mean you huffing and puffing while trying to show your son how to throw a ball or carrying your daughter up the stairs. You don't want to look back and think about all the games you could have played, if you'd only had the lungs for them.

The physical toll from alcohol can often be even worse, with 5.3% of deaths worldwide resulting from alcohol abuse. Beyond that, one in 10 children in the United States have an alcoholic parent; growing up in that environment can be a very tough situation. For the pregnancy, drinking may mean not being able to help out your spouse or missing important dates and events. Having a drink now and again is perfectly fine, but your priority should be your family. Although you don't need to cut these things out of your life completely, the effort in the long run will make you a better father, one that your kids will be able to look up to.

Emotional

It's not a guy's favorite subject, but having a kid means it's time for some introspection. Whether or not therapy is something you are interested in (it's person- ally helped me out a lot), you need to find a way to take stock of your emotional health. A stable man is a stable father, and you need to be sure you can keep an even keel when things get stressful. A little person will be depending on you now; some days, a lot of weight rests on your shoulders. Are you going to be able to keep your cool after being awake for 24 hours? Are you emotionally mature enough to be understanding when your wife experiences hormonal changes and may not be herself? There will be many situations that test your emotions, and you want to make sure you are internally prepared to meet those conflicts from a place of empathy.

You need to be strong, so you can help your wife be strong. Pregnancy can be a challenging time for a mother's mental health, and it's up to you to support her through that time in any way you can. I have learned that it takes a strong man to be able to do this successfully. While your feelings are still valid, part of going into this from a place of emotional strength means you may have to sacrifice your own happiness for a bit. Lose an argument, make concessions, compromise. Though a relationship is an equal partnership, the focus on pregnancy needs to be on your partner. But I promise it will all be worth it.

Fear #4: What will happen to them when I'm gone?

This can be an incredibly difficult thought to deal with. The reality is, the best possible scenario in life is that you pass before your child. In all likelihood, this is what will come to pass. You certainly wouldn't want it to be the other way around. So what will happen to them?

The truth is, you can't know. All you can do is take solace in having done your best to raise them. If you guide your child into adulthood and beyond, they should be ready to face life without you when your time comes. It can be scary, and your children will certainly miss you dearly, but you will get to live on through them, their children, and their children's children. Make sure to tell your children stories about your own parents and grandparents. By reminiscing on the memories of departed loved ones, you can create a tradition of passing family stories on to the next generation.

EACH MONTH WILL BRING SOMETHING NEW

So now that you've gotten some questions and worries out of the way, it's time to look forward to the future! With each chapter, your child will get a little bigger. Each month, there will be little changes, and medical terminology that can help you better understand what's happening. There will also be new challenges every month, and different methods for helping out your partner.

Let's start with the first month, when your child is so small they could sit on the *tip* of your finger.

LITTLE GRAIN OF RICE

"A Dad needs to show an incredible amount of respect, humor, and friendship toward his spouse, so the kids understand their parents are real people: they're fun, they do things together, they're best friends. Kids learn by example. If I respect Mom, they're going to respect Mom."

- Tim Allen, Famous TV Dad and Real-life Father

VOCABULARY FOR MONTH ONE:

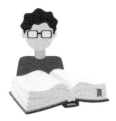

o·o·cyte

/ ōə sīt/

noun : BIOLOGY
An oocyte is a cell in an ovary which can undergo the process of meiotic division to form an ovum.

blas·to·cyst

/ blæstəʊ sɪst /

noun : EMBRYOL
A blastocyst is a distinctive stage of an embryo - a form of blastula that develops from a cluster of cells, the morula. A cavity appears in the morula between the cells of the inner cell mass and the enveloping layer. This cavity then becomes filled with fluid.

zy·gote

/ˈzī gōt/

Noun : BIOLOGY
A zygote is a diploid cell resulting from the fusion of two haploid gametes; a fertilized ovum.

te·rat·o·gen

/teˈradəjən/

Noun : BIOLOGY
plural noun: **teratogens**
A teratogen is an agent or factor which causes malformation of an embryo.

fal·lo·pi·an tube	pro·ges·ter·one
/fəˈlōpēən ˌtoōb/	/prōˈjestəˌrōn/
Noun BIOLOGY plural noun: **Fallopian tubes** The fallopian tubes are a pair of tube-like organs along which eggs travel from the ovaries to the uterus.	Noun BIOCHEMISTRY Progesterone is a steroid hormone released by the corpus luteum that stimulates the uterus to prepare for pregnancy.

em·bry·o	ec·top·ic preg·nan·cy
/ˈembrēˌō/	/ekˌtäpik ˈpregnənsē/
Noun EMBRYOL An embryo is an unborn offspring in the process of development, in particular a human offspring during the period from approximately the second to the eighth week after fertilization (after which it is usually termed a fetus).	Noun BIOLOGY An ectopic pregnancy is a pregnancy in which the fetus develops outside the uterus, typically in a fallopian tube.

THE FIRST MONTH

The first month of pregnancy begins three weeks after your partner's last menstrual cycle. It's usually within a few weeks of this point that couples find out they are pregnant. This can be because they are intentionally trying, and are taking tests regularly, or the woman begins to experience physical symptoms.

These physical symptoms can include:

- Missed Period: If your wife doesn't begin her menstrual cycle when it regularly occurs, that could indicate pregnancy. It isn't a guarantee though; every woman's cycle is different.
- Swollen or tender breasts: Hormonal changes early in pregnancy may cause a woman's breasts to become sore and sensitive. While this is a symptom your wife will likely experience throughout the next nine months, the discomfort will become more manageable as her body adjusts to the hormonal change.
- Nausea: The infamous morning sickness. Though more common further along into pregnancy, waves of nausea can occur within the first month. Also, morning sickness is a bit of a misnomer; I've personally had to hold Leah's hair back late at night. Be prepared for nausea at any time of the day!
- Frequent Urination: Increased frequency of urination is common throughout pregnancy, and can be an early indicator that someone is pregnant. A woman's body creates more bodily fluids during this time period, much of which must be processed by the kidneys. This extra processed liquid often ends up in the bladder.

- <u>Tiredness and Fatigue</u>: One of the most common early symptoms of pregnancy. A rise in the level of progesterone is often pinned as the culprit, though scientists haven't reached a consensus on the full cause of fatigue in early pregnancy.

One of the most important symptoms you need to be aware of is **mood swings.** Your partner's body is going to begin producing a flood of various hormones to help the baby grow. Not only that, but the stress of experiencing everything mentioned above can weigh on a person's mental health. This is where you need to draw from a well of empathy, one that you will be drinking from heavily over the next nine months. Try to understand what your wife is going through, and put yourself in her shoes. Especially since her feet might swell, and she might get sad when her feet don't fit into her favorite pair of sneakers.

Your partner may become:

- Angry
- Depressed
- Excited
- Anxious
- Overwhelmed
- Exhausted

Sometimes all at once. Understand her body is performing a miracle, but that miracle may cause a couple of biting comments. So here's some advice: try your best to avoid instigating or perpetuating unnecessary fights. You can win every argument after the baby is born, I promise. But for now, your partner is soaking in an evolutionary soup of hormones. Remember, they aren't trying to be mean or difficult, their body is under tremendous stress.

And never, and I mean never, say "Calm down." Once was enough for me.

Take this time to pamper your spouse with everything you know they love. Find a show or movie you both enjoy, one that is comedic and light if possible. Cook her favorite meal, or get take-out from a restaurant you know she enjoys. Let her know that everything is going to be alright, and you will be with her every step of the way.

WHAT SHOULD I DO FIRST?

First, you'll want to make an appointment with an OBGYN. OBGYN is an acronym: OB stands for obstetrician, a type of doctor who cares for women during childbirth and pregnancy. GYN stands for gynecologist, a doctor specializing in the female reproductive system.

This doctor will confirm the pregnancy and make sure that there are no initial complications. Check your health insurance plan to see that prenatal care is covered, so there are no financial surprises later on.

Next, I recommend keeping a baby diary. Obviously, I may have overdone it with my endless stack of journals, but a record of this time will be invaluable later. So much of the pregnancy will pass by in a blur, and it's great to be able to look back and see how you both were feeling, what you were doing, and what predictions you had about the future.

HEALTHY DIET

Now let's talk about diet. While your diet doesn't necessarily have to change, your wife certainly will. Personally, I recommend joining her: Not only will it show solidarity, but it will also save time and money. Why shop for two separate sets of food and cook two different dinners? A pregnancy diet won't do anything harmful to your body; it's an incredibly healthy way to eat.

First, make sure you provide a wide variety of fruits and vegetables. These will give your wife and the baby essential vitamins and nutrients, like folic acid and vitamin C. Folic acid supplements, usually 400mg a day, are also an excellent addition to the mother's diet, as these can significantly reduce the risk of congenital disabilities. Try to have a vegetable or a fruit with each meal. For example, you can have an orange at breakfast and a nice side of Brussel sprouts for dinner. Important note: Fruit does not mean fruit juice! Fruit juice often loses much of the nutrients of whole fruit and can include added sugar. It's always better to have fresh fruit when possible.

Next, you'll need lean protein. High-quality protein sources provide vitamin B, iron, and essential amino acids. Eggs are an excellent protein source, and you can hard boil them to create a healthy and easily accessible snack. Try to have protein with every meal; an example would be eggs with dinner, turkey on whole-grain bread for lunch, and a sliced chicken breast for dinner.

Carbs are often demonized in modern society, but some carbs have a lot of nutritional value. Whole grains like those found in rice, oatmeal, and whole-wheat bread can give you fiber, riboflavin, thiamin, and niacin. These aid in the absorption of other nutrients and help facilitate digestion.

Fat is another word we have associated with poor health, but healthy fats are absolutely vital to human function. They are one of the three primary macronutrients, the other two being carbohydrates and protein.

Almonds, avocados, walnuts, and fish are just some of the ways you can incorporate healthy fats into your diet. Fat helps give your body sustainable energy while supporting the organs and proper cell function. They also help increase the production of beneficial hormones.

Calcium is one of the most critical components in creating strong bones, and it can help boost nerve function and muscle activity. Dairy is a great way to get this nutrient, with products like cheese, milk, and yogurt providing a hefty dose of calcium. Yogurt makes a great snack to go along with that hard-boiled egg, and a glass of milk in the morning can help start the day off with bone-strengthening goodness.

The most important part of a pregnancy diet, or any diet for that matter, is **water.** Hydration is the cornerstone of a healthy body, whether that be a full-grown adult or a baby just beginning to grow in the womb. Most of the liquids you and your partner consume should be water, and if you can, try to get at least 8 cups of water per day. Have a refillable water bottle handy, preferably one that shows you how much you have drunk that day. It can be a chore at first, but once you feel how great it is to be hydrated, you'll bring that water bottle everywhere you go.

CHANGING HABITS

Certain activities have to be eliminated the moment a pregnancy has been confirmed. Smoking and drinking are two of the main ones: smoking while pregnant can cause birth defects, like a damaged heart and lungs. This damage can last into a baby's childhood and teen years, and can sometimes be permanent. Smoking will also slow your baby's growth and cause premature birth. Babies born prematurely can have many health issues, including problems with their brain, lungs, heart, eyes, and other organs.

Drinking has a similar host of adverse effects on pregnancy. Ingesting alcohol during pregnancy can increase your risk of miscarriage, premature birth, and low birthweight. It can also lead to fetal alcohol syndrome, a condition that results in brain damage and developmental issues. These issues can persist for a baby's entire life.

As the father, you are not required to quit. That being said, quitting along with your partner can be a massive morale boost. I abstained from drinking to be supportive during Leah's first pregnancy. Taking a break from drinking also allowed me to reassess my relationship with alcohol, and I found I had much more moderation once I began drinking again. Leah said the same thing; before the baby, she would usually have a single glass of wine with dinner most nights of the week. After the pregnancy and breastfeeding stage (where you also cannot drink), her drinking reduced to the occasional glass or two on special occasions.

Exercise will also become an important part of the pregnancy regiment. Staying active during pregnancy is proven to improve the health of both the mother and the baby. Experts recommend exercising at least three times a week for 30 minutes; this can improve blood flow, boost positive mood, and strengthen the heart and muscles. These workouts are not intended to be strenuous; taking a leisurely walk somewhere you can both get fresh air is my personal favorite couple's exercise. Make sure to purchase a comfortable pair of walking shoes and a good sports bra for your wife, and don't forget that water bottle! You want to make sure whatever form of exercise you choose poses no risk to your spouse. Now is not the time to enroll in your local hockey team or try mountain biking. Safety is crucial for you as well; an injury this early in the pregnancy could sideline you and reduce your ability to help your partner.

Another habit many forget is good sleep. Sleep, like water, is an essential component of a healthy, functioning body. If it's been a while, now might be the time to upgrade to a nicer bed. A white noise machine can often help someone get to sleep easier, along with aromatherapy candles (specifically lavender.) Remember that she will likely be wracked with fatigue and may be sleeping earlier and longer. Keep a regular sleep schedule so as not to disturb your wife, and do everything in your power to make sure she has a peaceful sleeping environment.

WHAT IS HAPPENING TO THE BABY DURING THE FIRST MONTH?

The process of pregnancy starts with fertilization, as a single sperm will dive into an egg to create a zygote. This zygote begins to divide and will become an embryo. This embryo will then travel down the fallopian tubes and attach to the uterine wall. During the first month, your spouse may notice a light spotting of blood. This means that the embryo has attached to the wall of her uterus. This process will take several days, and once the attachment is successful, the pregnancy has officially begun. If a person does not become pregnant, they will have a period, which sheds the uterine lining and the embryo along with it.

At this point, the baby will be about 1/6th of an inch long and begin to develop their head and torso. The beginning structure of their arms and legs, called limb buds, will appear. The brain will start to grow in several areas, with cranial nerves beginning to be visible. Ears and eyes will begin to form, along with tissue that will develop into their skeletal system. The heart will also develop, and blood will start to flow through the main vessels.

MISCARRIAGE

One of the most difficult subjects to discuss is, of course, miscarriage. A miscarriage is when an embryo or fetus dies before the 20th week of pregnancy. The risk of miscarriage is far higher in the initial stage of pregnancy, with 10-15 percent of all pregnancies ending prematurely, with 8 out of 10 of those miscarriages occurring in the first three months.

A common myth is that miscarriages often happen due to the actions of the pregnant person, but this is simply not true. Everyday activities like exercise, working, sex, or regular ingestion of medications do not cause miscarriage. Even minor injuries like falling rarely cause a miscarriage. Often, what causes a miscarriage is random chance. If the fertilized egg has an abnormal number of chromosomal genes, a miscarriage can occur. Some illnesses or infections can also cause a loss of the child, along with abnormalities in the uterus. You can talk to your OBGYN about tests to see if any of these risk factors apply to your spouse.

You can take specific steps to lower your chance of experiencing a miscarriage, many of which we have already discussed in this chapter.

These steps include:

- Eating a healthy diet
- Avoiding unnecessary medications
- Exercising on a regular basis
- Taking special care of your spouse's abdomen
- Talking to your doctor about what over-the-counter drugs can be taken
- Understanding and managing stress
- Abstaining from nicotine and alcohol
- Avoiding unclean environments to reduce the risk of infections

Even if you take all these precautions, a miscarriage may still occur. This can be an incredibly challenging experience to go through, and don't hesitate to seek out therapeutic assistance for you and your spouse. Work with your health care provider to understand what happened, and if you are ready, plan a future pregnancy.

FROM RICE TO RASPBERRY

As the first month ends and the second month begins, your baby will continue to grow. As with the first month, you will encounter new challenges and developments, but you'll notice that some of your fear has begun to subside. The first month is one of the hardest: while you are doing everything you can for your partner, you are also wrestling with your own worries and anxieties about the future. Once you start to really get into the pregnancy, there will be plenty to focus on. For now, let's take a look at what you can expect in the second month.

3

LITTLE RASPBERRY

"Am I the Raddest, Baddest Dad a Kid Ever Had?"

- Bob Saget, as Danny Tanner on Full House

VOCABULARY FOR MONTH TWO:

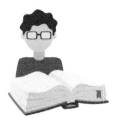

cer·vix

/ˈsərviks/

noun : BIOLOGY

The cervix is the narrow passage forming the lower end of the uterus.

chro·mo·some

/ˈkrōməˌsōm/

noun BIOLOGY

A chromosome is a threadlike structure of nucleic acids and protein. They are found in the nucleus of most living cells, and carry genetic information in the form of genes.

dop·pler ma·chine

/ˈdäplər məˈSHēn/

noun MEDICINE

A Doppler machine is used to perform a doppler ultrasound, a noninvasive ultrasound test that estimates the blood flow through your blood vessels. The procedure does this by bouncing high-frequency sound waves off circulating red blood cells. Unlike a regular ultrasound, which also uses sound waves to produce images, a doppler machine can show blood flow.

hy·per·em·e·sis gra·vi·dar·um

/hīpəˈreməsəs graˈvuhˈdehˈruhm/

noun MEDICINE

Hyperemesis gravidarum is the medical term for severe nausea and vomiting during pregnancy. The symptoms can be severely uncomfortable. You might vomit more than four times a day, become dehydrated, feel constantly dizzy and lightheaded and lose ten pounds or more.

hu·man cho·ri·on·ic go·nad·o·tro·pin

/ (h)yo͞omən kôrē änik gō nadə trōpən/

noun : EMBRYOL

Human chorionic gonadotropin, or HCG, is a hormone produced in the human placenta that maintains the corpus luteum during pregnancy. These levels peak in your first trimester, then gradually decline for the remainder of your pregnancy.

em·bry·on·ic tail

/ embrē änik tāl/

noun : EMBRYOL

The embryonic tail usually grows into the coccyx or the tailbone. The tailbone is a bone located at the end of the spine, below the sacrum. Sometimes, however, the embryonic tail doesn't disappear and the baby is born with it. This is a true human tail. Growing a true human tail is extremely rare.

car·ti·lage

/ kärdlij/

noun ANATOMY

Firm, whitish, flexible connective tissue found in various forms in the larynx and respiratory tract, in structures such as the external ear, and in the articulating surfaces of joints. It is more widespread in the infant skeleton, being replaced by bone during growth.

cra·ni·um

/ krānēəm/

noun ANATOMY

The cranium is the medical term for the skull, specifically the part enclosing the brain.

im·plan·ta·tion bleed·ing

/ implan tāSH(ə)n blēdiNG/

noun MEDICINE

Implantation bleeding is defined as the small amount of spotting or bleeding that occurs about 10 to 14 days after conception. This occurrence is considered normal. The cause of implantation bleeding is thought to happen when the fertilized egg attaches to the lining of the uterus.

fe·tus

/ fēdəs/

noun BIOLOGY

A developmental stage of an unborn child, specifically a baby eight weeks after conception.

THE SECOND MONTH

By the second month, you'll start to settle into the reality of your approaching fatherhood. Keeping busy helps ease the transition, and there is always plenty to do. The second month will involve a continuation of certain pregnancy side effects, new kinds of doctor visits, and new developments for the baby.

Your first official pregnancy visit should happen this month, and you will have regular appointments once a month until the end of the pregnancy. The doctor will likely ask your partner about their personal and family medical history, their current health, and any risk factors they may face in their day-to-day activities. The doctor will likely run a series of tests to complete their full assessment.

These tests will likely include:

- Pap Smear: A pap smear, sometimes referred to as a pap test, is a cervical examination intended to detect the presence of cancer. Cells are collected from inside of the cervix and tested to see if the patient has cervical cancer. Pap smears are a safe procedure for pregnant women and have not been connected to miscarriage. There can be some blood that accompanies a pap smear, but that is due to increased blood flow to the uterus and cervix.

- Pelvic Examination: A pelvic exam is a procedure designed to evaluate a woman's reproductive organs. The doctor can confirm the pregnancy, assess the health of the vagina, cervix, and pelvic bones, as well as check for cysts. This test helps find possible future complications early in the pregnancy and is usually conducted again at around 36 weeks.
- Urine and Blood Tests: Urine and blood tests serve several purposes for pregnant women, including confirming the pregnancy. Doctors do this by checking for high levels of HCG, a hormone made by the placenta during pregnancy, in the woman's blood and urine. These tests will also look for the presence of protein (which may indicate kidney problems) and sugar (which may be a sign of diabetes). Your doctor may also run auxiliary blood tests to check for iron levels, disease immunities, and any possible infections that may complicate the pregnancy.
- Height and Weight: A standard procedure for most doctor's appointments, height will not be especially important to the pregnancy. Weight gain generally doesn't happen until later in the

pregnancy, with 1 to 5 pounds being the norm. Some women even report losing weight, often due to their feelings of nausea.

- Blood Pressure: Blood pressure is measured to establish a baseline and monitored throughout pregnancy. A healthy blood pressure reading should be below 120/80, but not so low that a person develops low blood pressure. Both high and low come with their own set of symptoms and complications, but your doctor can recommend a treatment regimen to deal with either.

- Abdominal Examination: An examination of the abdomen will take place to assess the position of the fundus or the area at the top of the uterus. Fundal height, or the distance between the top of the uterus and the pubic bone, will increase later in pregnancy. The doctor will take a baseline measurement now to assess the height change later on.

Most of these tests will form the foundation for the pregnancy's medical record, and your doctor will add subsequent examinations and test results as the months go on. You can ask your doctor for a copy of these records, which can come in handy if you ever need medical care from a different provider.

This first appointment is an excellent opportunity to ask any of those burning questions you've been having. Take the time to discuss with your partner beforehand what information you would like, and a doctor should be happy to provide the answers. Make sure to have your partner jot down any symptoms they are having, a list of their medications and supplements, and any other information the doctor may need. You'll also want to plan future appointments here. Dealing with scheduling can be a hassle, and you don't want the stress of making an appointment last minute. See how far out you can get on your doctor's calendar, so you have one less thing to worry about.

A doctor may also ask if your spouse would like a nuchal translucency measurement test. This procedure involves an ultrasound that measures the fluid space on the back of your baby's neck. These results, along with your spouse's age and hormone levels, can determine what risk your baby has of a chromosomal abnormality. These tests are no guarantee of a confirmed diagnosis, but can allow your doctor to run subsequent tests to find any abnormalities. With more information about your baby's chromosomes, you can better prepare for any developmental issues that may occur.

SYMPTOMS IN MONTH TWO

Many of the symptoms your wife experienced in the previous months will persist, most noticeably her **morning sickness**. It's important not to get frustrated here, as you will likely be woken up at least once a night so your partner can run to the bathroom. Having a bucket near the bed may not be the prettiest solution, but it can help in case of an emergency.

There are a couple of things you can do to help your partner's morning sickness, like:

- Keep Fresh Foods On Hand: While your spouse may seek out comfort foods, this can actually make their nausea worse. Greasy foods like french fries, spicy foods like peppers, and fatty foods like cheeseburgers are more challenging to digest. While it's not very fun, bland foods like bananas, toast, and rice are far easier to stomach. Smaller meals or snacks throughout the day also help keep the stomach less full, which can help ease the digestion process.
- Water, Water and...*Water*: We've discussed the general importance of water, but good fluid intake can also help with the symptoms of nausea. It also helps keep something in the stomach, as dry heaves can be very painful. If

your partner is growing tired of water, you can try adding a sugar-free flavoring or substituting the occasional glass of ginger ale.

- Fresh Air: One of the great benefits of taking walks and getting your daily exercise is that sweet fresh air. The cool temperatures and plentiful oxygen of being outdoors can help counteract the hypothalamus's quest to raise body temperature, one of the leading forces behind nausea.

- Nausea Triggers: Being observant and noticing what generally precipitates a bout of morning sickness can help you identify nausea triggers. These triggers can be certain foods, a particular smell, or quick movement. Keep a list of what generally sends your spouse running for the toilet, and do your best to keep these items away from her throughout the pregnancy.

- Rinse and Repeat: Your partner will want to rinse her mouth after each instance of vomiting. One reason for this is the lingering taste can increase her nausea symptoms. Another would be that the acid from your stomach can damage your teeth, melting the enamel. After losing your lunch, a good way to rinse is to wash out the mouth with water mixed with a teaspoon of baking soda. Baking soda is very base, so it can neutralize the acid.

- Vitamins and Natural Remedies: Taking prenatal vitamins by themselves can make a person feel queasy, so it's best to take them with a light snack and a small cup of water. Natural remedies can help here too, and fresh ginger or a ginger supplement can help soothe the stomach.

Bleeding

A common symptom that will begin to rear its head during the second month is vaginal bleeding. Medical experts have estimated that between 20% to 30% of all women will experience bleeding in the first trimester, which often causes distress. Make sure to reassure your partner that this is entirely normal. When a fertilized egg implants in the uterus, a normal process called implantation bleeding occurs. The cervix may also bleed, particularly if you engage in sexual activity. The cervix can bleed so easily because it becomes incredibly sensitive during pregnancy and may bleed at the slightest touch.

If the bleeding is causing concern or becomes heavy or frequent, it's essential to contact your doctor. Bleeding can be a sign of miscarriage, and you'll want to find out what's happening quickly.

EMOTIONAL CHANGES

Many different factors can affect your partner's emotions this month. Between physical symptoms and hormonal changes, always be prepared for a sudden shift in mood. Upset to elated to angry, remind yourself this is all very normal. The hormones needed to create a baby are incredibly powerful and rather miraculous, so it's really no surprise that they take a toll on the person creating the child. Do what you can to ease this burden. Comfort your partner when they voice concerns about the pregnancy, whether that be a single glass of wine they had before a doctor fully confirmed the pregnancy, fears they may lose the child to miscarriage, or worries about sticking to new diets and medical regimens.

Damage to your partner's self-esteem can also become an issue as your wife may worry about potential weight gain, making her less attractive. Remind her that you'll love her no matter what, and that weight gain is often less of a factor than commonly thought. Regular exercise will help here, both with emotional regulation and keeping off unwanted pounds. Romance is an important factor to keep up here as well: remind your wife how special and beautiful she is by continuing to take her out to (healthy) dinners, a funny movie, or a moonlit walk through the park. It can be hard to find time after the baby has been born to make the time for romantic endeavors, and you should cherish the alone time you have with your spouse. Don't hyperfocus on your upcoming role as a father and forget your role as a lover. Never stop dating your spouse, and let them know how much they mean to you every day.

CHANGES IN SEX DRIVE

Certain aspects of your physical relationship will change over the course of the pregnancy. For example, a woman's interest in sex can change drastically, whether that be an increase or a decrease in sex drive. The most likely outcome for many pregnancies is a combination of both. Depending on what stage of the pregnancy your spouse is in, their sex drive will probably fluctuate.

In the first trimester, your spouse is more likely to have a decrease in sex drive. This decreased sex drive is often caused by hormonal changes, like raised progesterone levels. Increased progesterone can reduce sexual desire, not to mention causing the physical symptoms we discussed before, like fatigue and nausea. Someone experiencing the adverse effects of a new pregnancy for the first time may not feel well enough to have sex, and that's perfectly normal. However, as these hormones taper off around the 10th week, a pregnant woman's sex drive often returns.

At this stage, increased blood flow can make certain parts of your partner's body more sensitive, like the breasts, vulva, and sexual organs. This increased sensitivity can mean that touch may be difficult, but it can also cause easier arousal; this is a good thing! If your partner wishes to have sex, and you are also in the mood, it can be a great way to strengthen your bond and keep the romance alive. It's also great to take these moments while you can. Believe me, finding time to yourselves may be difficult once the baby has arrived.

WHAT IS HAPPENING TO THE BABY DURING THE SECOND MONTH?

At the beginning of month two, your child will be about ½ of an inch in length or about the size of a raspberry. By the end of the month, the baby will grow to a full inch in length (1/30 of an ounce), but you really won't notice much change in your spouse's stomach. A slight baby bump might appear, but she won't really start to show until the second trimester.

On the other hand, your baby is going through a variety of changes. These changes include:

- Changing from a curled posture to a more stretched out, lengthened one
- The embryonic tail, which grows initially on the coccyx, will likely be gone by the eighth week of the pregnancy
- The baby's closed eyes, which begin on the sides of their cranium, will slowly move to their permanent position on the front of their head
- The development of the nose and jaw will continue, defining the shape of your baby's face
- The beginnings of their arms, legs, fingers, and toes
- Soft bone begins to replace cartilage
- The detection of a heartbeat, usually at around six weeks
- Twenty tiny teeth will begin to bud within the gums by week 10
- Development of the palate and vocal cords
- Near completion of vital organ systems, including:

    - Central nervous system
    - Spinal cord
    - Neural tissue

- ○ Sensory organs
- ○ Digestive tract

- The left and right hemispheres of the brain will be fully formed, with brain cell mass growing at a rapid pace
- The liver will begin to create red blood cells, a job which bone marrow will take over in the third trimester

FROM RASPBERRY TO FIG

As the second month comes to an end, take a look over your journals. See what questions you had in that first month, and decide whether you've found conclusive answers to your queries. Write down new questions you've had more recently, and jot down your thoughts and feelings. As we transition into the third month, several things will get easier. First, the fear of miscarriage begins to dissipate, as the chances of this happening after the 3rd month are drastically lower. The baby will start to develop more rapidly, and you can start deciding whether you want to know the sex early or not. Certain challenges will arise, but I'm sure you'll be able to meet them. Let's take a look at what you can expect in month three.

4

LITTLE FIG

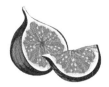

"No matter how big you get, you'll always be my son."

- Goofy to his son Max, as Bill Farmer in A Goofy Movie

VOCABULARY FOR MONTH THREE:

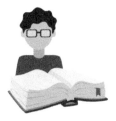

um·bil·i·cal cord

/ˌəmˈbilək(ə)l ˌkôrd/

*noun*BIOLOGY
A flexible cordlike structure containing blood vessels and attaching a human or other mammalian fetus to the placenta during gestation.

la·maze

/ləˈmäz/

*adjective*BIRTHING
Lamaze is a method of childbirth that involves exercises and breathing control. It is meant to give pain relief to a mother without the use of drugs.

chor·i·on·ic vill·us samp·ling

/chor·aɪ·ɒn·ic vill·ʌs sæmp·lɪŋ/

noun MEDICINE
Chorionic villus sampling, or CVS, is a prenatal test involving a tissue sample taken from the placenta. This sample is assessed to determine if the child may have chromosomal abnormalities or other genetic problems.

pla·cen·ta

/pləˈsen(t)ə/

*noun*BIOLOGY
A flattened circular organ in the uterus of pregnant eutherian mammals, nourishing and maintaining the fetus through the umbilical cord.

yolk sac

/yōk sak/

*noun*BIOLOGY
A yolk sac is a sac lacking yolk in the early embryo of a mammal.

gin·gi·vi·tis

/ˌjinjəˈvīdəs/

*noun*MEDICINE
Gingivitis is a dental disease involving inflammation of the gums.

fa·tigue	am·ni·ot·ic flu·id
/fə ˈtēg/	/ˌamnē ˌädik ˈflo͞oid/
*noun*MEDICINE	*noun*BIOLOGY
Fatigue is a medical condition involving extreme tiredness, usually resulting from mental or physical exertion or illness.	Amniotic fluid is the fluid surrounding a fetus within the amnion.

THE THIRD MONTH

In the final month of the first trimester, you'll start to settle into the flow of things. Managing doctors appointments, helping to relieve pregnancy symptoms, providing quality foods; all of these will begin to be second nature. Certain ailments your partner is dealing with will subside, and others may pop up. Certain fears, like miscarriage, become much less likely. Overall, the third month can be where a bit of that initial stress goes away.

This is a good time to schedule a dentist appointment. Pregnant women are more susceptible to inflamed gums and gingivitis, and it's best to prevent these conditions before they begin. Regular cleanings and dentist check-ups can look for the warning signs of these dental conditions, and save you money in costly procedures down the road.

Now is also the time to make a decision on finding out the sex of the baby. An ultrasound can determine the baby's sex as early as 14 weeks, so you should have a conversation about whether you want the reveal to be a surprise. While this is a romantic idea, it can make certain preparations more difficult. Knowing the sex allows you to buy items for either your baby boy or girl. While many toys and clothes are unisex, it can still help to know ahead of time what sex to expect.

SYMPTOMS IN MONTH THREE

Many of the symptoms your spouse has been dealing with will continue, especially nausea. Make sure to review the tips from the previous chapter under "Symptoms in Month Two". That being said, there will be new issues popping up during this month. Here is a list of the symptoms your partner may be experiencing during month three.

- Vaginal discharge: The hormones produced during pregnancy, along with the increased blood supply to help the baby's growth, will likely lead to an increase in vaginal discharge. This is completely normal, and as long as your spouse doesn't detect anything abnormal about the discharge (e.g. a bad or unhealthy smell) there is nothing to worry about; if there is concern you can talk with your doctor. There isn't much you can do to assist with this symptom: purchasing breathable undergarments can help prevent infection, and make your partner more comfortable.

- Frequent urination: Carrying a little one means that space within the body can start to get cramped. With more pressure on the bladder, trips to the bathroom may become a frequent and tedious chore. Increased fluid intake, while completely necessary, isn't making it any easier. Make sure to know the location of a bathroom anywhere you go, so your partner doesn't have to worry about dealing with a full bladder.

- Headaches: While headaches can occur during all trimesters, and often for different reasons, those that occur most often first, are tension headaches. Your partner may feel a dull ache, or a pulsating throb on the sides of their head. Headaches can aggravate nausea, and overall make your spouse very uncomfortable. While you want to check with your primary care doctor before taking any medication during pregnancy, it is generally safe for pregnant women to take over-the-counter headache medicine. This includes medication like advil, where the active ingredient is acetaminophen.

- Breast growth and tenderness: During the third month your spouse will begin to notice their breasts growing in size. This can be accompanied by a tender feeling, and even pain when touched. You may need to help your spouse shop for bras specifically for the pregnancy, and help find low-impact exercises to avoid irritating the more tender areas.

- Constipation: Hormonal changes can affect the speed of the digestive system, and cause constipation. Some of the prenatal vitamins may also aggravate this problem, specifically iron supplements. Make sure your spouse stays hydrated, and try to introduce more fiber into their diet. Vegetables, fresh fruit, and whole grain foods are a good way to add fiber naturally.

- Fatigue and trouble sleeping: These two symptoms go hand in hand, as difficulty sleeping at night can make someone fatigued the following day. Your partner's body is diverting a massive amount of energy and nutrients to the baby, and draining the resources available for their own needs. With the baby bump developing, it can be difficult to sleep in certain positions. Make sure to keep up the exercise routine, as this can help reduce fatigue and increase sleep quality. Make sure to maintain good sleep hygiene as well; try to make your bed an area just for sleep. Reduce the use of devices near bed time, as these emit sleep-damaging blue light.

- Dizziness: That same sapping of nutrients can also mean that feelings of dizziness may occur. You want to make sure snacks are never far from reach, along with a cold glass of water. Low blood sugar can lead to dizziness, with dehydration contributing to symptoms of light-headedness. Something healthy like mixed nuts, and a comfortable chair to sit down in, can help her deal with these dizzy spells.

- Changes in Skin: During pregnancy, your body produces a type of pigment called melanin in much higher amounts. This extra pigmentation can cause brown patches on the skin called chloasma. These patches can occur on the face, or as a long vertical line running from the pubic area to the belly button. Again, this is totally normal, and your spouse has nothing to worry about. Most of these changes in skin color will disappear by the time your baby is born.

- Forgetfulness (also known as "pregnancy brain"): With the combination of sleep deprivation, hormonal changes, and stress, many pregnant women experience a symptom colloquially known as "pregnancy brain". These are minor periods of forgetfulness, where a person may have small lapses in short-term memory. Pregnancy brain has also been described as a sort of fog, and can be incredibly frustrating for your partner. Overall, watch for the following symptoms to identify if pregnancy brain may be happening:

  o Poor concentration
  o Clumsiness
  o Absentmindness
  o Disorientation
  o Difficulty reading
  o Difficulty recalling words or names

The best thing you can do for your spouse is reduce the stress causing these memory issues. If they seem to be having trouble finding an item or recalling information, gently help them find what they are looking for. If they are getting frustrated, go out of your way to relieve that frustration. A nice bubble bath is my go to, with a couple of candles and calming music to set the mood.

BIRTHING CLASSES

Reading is a great way to educate yourself, but some subjects are better learned in a hands-on environment. Birthing classes are a good way to talk with certified experts about various techniques and methods for childbirth. You can also meet other soon-to-be parents, learn from their pregnancy experiences, and even offer some advice of your own. Let's look at three methods often taught in birthing classes, and their different advantages.

Lamaze Method

You've likely heard of the Lamaze method, and for good reason; it's an incredibly popular technique that's been used by countless women in childbirth. The Lamaze method was designed to remind parents that childbirth is a natural event. The environment of a hospital can make the process feel a bit alien; with the Lamaze method, you and your partner will be shown how to approach childbirth with less stress and more familiarity.

The method is named for its creator, a French obstetrician named Ferdinand Lamaze. The Lamaze method began to grow in popularity in the late 50's, with classes popping up all over the United States. The stated goal of the Lamaze Method is simple: To increase women's confidence in their birthing ability. The program accomplishes this through several central components.

1. Unless there are medical complications, allow labor to begin on its own.
2. Birthing moms should have support during labor, whether that be from a partner, friend, or family member.
3. Labor is not a rigid procedure; women should move around, change positions, and even walk during labor. If possible, don't give birth on your back.
4. Medical interventions should only occur when necessary
5. Women are encouraged to follow their bodies natural urges to push.
6. After the birth, the mother and baby should be kept together.

A Lamaze class usually involves groups of 6 to 12 couples meeting for a total of 12 hours. Each class lasts between one to two hours. These classes can include:

- Watching birthing videos

- Instructions on how to be active and informed during both labor and birth
- The breathing techniques to use during labor
- Natural coping mechanisms for labor pain, including walking, position changes, massage, and hydrotherapy
- How to get the most out of professional support during labor and birth
- Partner tips for labor and birth support
- How to communicate during labor and birth
- Complications that can occur during labor and birth, and the medical interventions that will help
- Pain management, including information about epidurals and other medication
- How to interact with your baby after birth
- Initial breastfeeding

Bradley Technique

The Bradley technique of childbirth preparation is another popular option for parents looking for alternative birthing experiences. Created in 1947 by Dr. Robert Bradley, the purpose of the program was to design a way to support women through labor and birth without the use of medication. While the method does allow for medical intervention in the case of an emergency, it encourages as natural of a birth as possible.

Besides a lack of medication or medical intervention, the Bradley method is built on several central tenets. These guidelines are generally conducted by the labor-coach, which would most likely be you. You'll need to complete these steps to make sure the labor and birth go as smoothly as possible.

1. *Low-light environment:* While many hospitals require bright lights to conduct procedures, Dr. Bradley believes that pregnant women need a less harsh environment for birth.
2. *Privacy:* While a woman in labor shouldn't be alone, nobody wants a crowd. Dr. Bradley says that the only ones in the labor room should be those that are absolutely necessary. This means their partner or another person with a close relationship to the mother.
3. *Complete Comfort:* The mother should be as comfortable as possible so they can focus on the labor process. This means if the room is too hot, it needs to be cooled down. If your partner is sweating, dab the sweat from their face. Anything you can do to increase comfort and reduce stress should be done.

4. *A Feeling of Safety:* Your partner should feel 100% safe in the birthing environment, and as their labor coach you need to establish this safety. If any concerns should arise, let your partner know you have it handled and they are safe under your care.

5. *Familiarity With Surroundings:* The birthing place should be, if possible, somewhere familiar to the mother. That means at home, a trusted friend's house, or in another safe place. If the birth must take place at a hospital, try to visit the facility beforehand to establish that familiarity.

6. *Confidence:* Dr. Bradley believes that the mother must be completely confident in her drug-free birthing decision. He says that the need for medication is an expectation created by society, and if a woman does not believe she can do it, labor will be more difficult.

7. *Relaxation:* One of the most important parts of the Bradley method is relaxation. Tension can make labor pains excruciating, and relaxation can help move the birthing process along more quickly. This is the reason that position changes are encouraged; your partner should find what makes her most comfortable during labor, and move around freely.

8. *Natural And Controlled Breathing:* Dr. Bradley says that the mother should try to imitate the calm breathing patterns of sleep, and focus on stress-free control. Women are encouraged to focus on their breathing as a distraction from the pain of labor.

9. *Mother-Baby Bonding:* After the birth, the Bradley method encourages the mother to put the baby on her breast immediately. This helps bond the mother and child, and warm the baby post-birth.

At a Bradley technique class, you will learn a wide variety of information about all facets of childbirth. This information can include:

- How a natural birth works
- The risks involved with medical intervention
- The best prenatal nutrition
- Techniques for relaxation
- Safe prenatal exercises for birth preparation
- How to be a birthing coach
- Labor and delivery positions
- How to bond with and breastfeed an infant
- Basic care of an infant
- How to create the best birthing environment
- Encouragement tips during labor and birth

Hypnobirthing

A popular choice among celebrities, hypnobirthing is a technique that involves the use of hypnosis for pain management and labor facilitation. The method was created in 1989 by hypnotherapist Marie Mongan, and aims to give a non-medical option to women who are worried about the birth and labor process. Hypnobirthing is designed to not only help with pain, but put the mother in a relaxed state so the natural birthing process can take place.

The method involves three main components to help the mother get into a hypnotic state: **Positivity**, **Visualization**, and **Controlled Breathing**.

Positivity

Hypnobirthing puts a large focus on creating a positive environment for the mother during labor and birth. This includes changing certain words to have a softer feeling and more positive connotation. For example, a word like "contraction" would become something like a "wave". This can help put the mother in a better mindset, making the process much easier to handle. I can say firsthand that these word changes made a world of a difference for Leah. I highly recommend this.

Visualization

The hypnotherapist will provide guided visualization, and help the mother find a meditative state during birth. This involves having your spouse picture a place that relaxes them, or an event that puts them at ease. Finding a "happy place" as it were helps distract from pain and relax your spouse during labor.

Controlled Breathing

There are two techniques for breathing in hypno-birthing: "four count" and "seven count". In "four count", your partner will breathe in and out of their nose. They will breathe in for four seconds, and out for seven seconds. In "seven count", your partner will breathe in the same manner, but for seven seconds in and out. This breathing pattern is meant to activate the parasympathetic nervous system, and lower stress levels.

WHAT IS HAPPENING TO THE BABY DURING THE THIRD MONTH?

By the conclusion of the third trimester, your child will be about 3-4 inches in length and weigh around 1 ounce. At this point, all of your child's organs will be present. Some may be at different developmental stages, but in technical terms, your baby is fully formed.

Your baby will have feet, toes, arms, hands, and fingers as well; they will begin to move slightly, but your partner won't be able to feel those famous "kicks" quite yet.

The membrane over the mouth between your baby and the amniotic fluid will begin to disappear, and the bowels will begin to lengthen. Although the digestive system is forming rapidly, it won't yet have any function. The pancreas, gallbladder, and liver will also begin to bud during this time. The tube that will become the rectum will divide from the gut, and begin to form the bladder and urethra on the front.

FROM FIG TO LEMON

As we move from the first to second trimester, your baby's growth will begin to increase exponentially. Different areas of your partner's body will experience changes to accommodate this growth, and the process can be painful. In month number four, there will be ailments your partner experiences that need your attention. You'll also begin to see a noticeable baby bump, which can be an exciting mile marker! Alright Dad, let's take a look at what you can expect in the beginning of the second trimester.

5

LITTLE LEMON

"We're gonna love the baby, we're gonna raise the baby to believe that anything is possible..."

- John Goodman, as Dan Connor on Rosanne

VOCABULARY FOR MONTH FOUR:

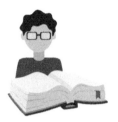

ges·ta·tion
/jeˈstāSH(ə)n/

*noun*BIOLOGY
Gestation is the process of carrying or being carried in the womb between conception and birth. The "gestational age" is a term used to describe how far along a pregnancy is.

u·ri·nal·y·sis
/ˌyo͝orəˈnaləsəs/

*noun*MEDICINE
Urinalysis is a medical procedure involving analysis of urine by physical, chemical, and microscopical means to test for the presence of disease, drugs, etc.

GERD
/gərd/

*noun*MEDICINE
Short for gastroesophageal reflux disease, GERD is a disease in which stomach acid or bile irritates the food pipe lining.

fun·dal height
/ˈfəndal hīt/

*noun*MEDICINE
Fundal height, or McDonald's rule, is a measure of the size of the uterus used to assess fetal growth and development during pregnancy. It is measured from the top of the mother's uterus to the top of the mother's pubic symphysis.

mid·wife	food crav·ing
/ˈmidˌwīf/	/fo͞od ˈkrāviNG/
*noun*MEDICINE	*noun*BIOLOGY
A midwife is a person (typically a woman) trained to assist women in childbirth.	A food craving is an intense desire for a specific food. This desire can seem uncontrollable, and a person may feel as though they cannot satisfy their hunger until they get that particular food.

es·tro·gen	tes·tos·ter·one
/ˈestrəjən/	/teˈstästəˌrōn/
*noun*BIOLOGY	*noun*BIOLOGY
Estrogen is defined as any of a group of steroid hormones which promote the development and maintenance of female characteristics of the body. Such hormones are also produced artificially for use in oral contraceptives or to treat menopausal and menstrual disorders.	Testosterone is a steroid hormone that stimulates development of male secondary sexual characteristics, produced mainly in the testes, but also in the ovaries and adrenal cortex.

THE FOURTH MONTH

As the second trimester begins, your spouse will notice some positive changes in her pregnancy symptoms. One great change about entering month four: less morning sickness! Your partner's nausea, while not disappearing entirely, should begin to taper off a bit as you enter the 14th week. The fatigue she felt should also become less prominent, and you may find yourself walking further and further on your daily exercise excursions. These are both due to a stabilization of hormones, which will also reduce the appearance of moodswings and reinvigorate your partner's sex drive. Overall, many uncomfortable symptoms will become less of a hassle during this period.

Not everything will be sunshine and rainbows, unfortunately. As you enter month four, new symptoms will begin to arise. Some of these will have to do with the development of the famous "baby bump". While there is nothing wrong with the appearance of a baby belly, there are some associated ailments that accompany your child's rapid increase in growth. None of these are too dire, but still require attention so your partner can be as comfortable as possible.

THE BABY BUMP

The appearance of the baby bump will be when many people, even strangers, begin to ask questions that are a bit too personal. Whether it be "how far along are you", "is it going to be a girl or a boy", or "can I touch it", it's normal for your partner to be a bit annoyed with the inquisition. Talk to your partner about their boundaries, and be ready to slap someone's hand away if they try to rub her belly for good luck.

What the baby bump really means is that your child is getting to a significant size. While the uterus is designed to expand and accomodate a child, the body will still start to feel a bit cramped. Your partner may even feel the first signs of a movement; these feelings can often manifest as a butterfly-like fluttering in the stomach. But along with that fluttering comes a laundry list of new symptoms:

- Abdominal Pain: As your baby grows, so does your partner's uterus. To make room, the ligaments in the uterus will stretch to support the expanded space. This stretching can cause dull pains in the lower abdomen, and even the occasional sharp stab. When this problem arises, help your partner find a position that makes them feel more comfortable. Moving around can adjust the position of the uterus, so your spouse can find a spot that doesn't cause any aches or pains.
- Heartburn and GERD: Uterine expansion often means the uterus will rise into the abdomen. This, along with pregnancy hormones relaxing stomach valves and releasing stomach acid into the esophagus, will cause heartburn. If this happens frequently, your partner may be suffering from GERD, also known as acid-reflux. You can help the symptoms of GERD

with several small behavioral changes,
including:

○ Smaller meals

○ Eating slowly

○ Avoiding trigger foods and drinks, like those
that are high in greasy fats, spice, filled with
citrus, caffeinated, or carbonated

○ Try not to eat for a minimum of three hours
before bed

○ Elevate your head during sleep

○ Try not to lay down after meals

There are also medications you can take, but every
pregnancy is different. Make sure to talk to your doctor
about what medicine is safe for your partner to take.

- Nasal congestion: Extra blood is needed to help
  fill the new blood vessels in your partner's baby
  bump. This increased volume, along with
  changes in hormones, can cause the mucus
  membranes of the nose to swell and congest.
  This congestion can even lead to bleeding if it
  gets out of hand. Give your partner saline nasal
  drops, and make sure they are hydrated. A
  humidifier can also help, and be turned on at
  night to make sleep-breathing easier.

- <u>Stretch marks</u>: As the stomach grows, the skin will stretch. This can lead to small skin changes called stretch marks. Stretch marks are completely normal, and there isn't a way to prevent them from occurring during pregnancy. You can help your partner moisturize to reduce the itchiness and irritation that can accompany these marks. Make sure to also reassure them if they are worried, as many of these stretch marks will disappear after the baby is born.

- <u>Spider veins</u>: Often appearing as red or purple networks of veins, spider veins are a similar occurrence to varicose veins. Circulatory pathways change during pregnancy, and this adjustment of blood flow can cause slight damage to some of your partner's veins. Again, this is completely normal, and most spider veins will disappear shortly after the baby's birth.

FOOD CRAVINGS

Food cravings will occur throughout the pregnancy, but you'll start to see a serious increase in the second trimester. As the baby needs more nutrients to grow, your spouse will likely begin to want strange and plentiful snacks. The most common snacks mothers request include:

- Sweets, like desserts and candy
- Meats, like beef, chicken, and pork
- Carbohydrate-heavy foods like pizza
- Fruits like strawberries and mangoes

You may also notice that your partner will turn their nose up at foods they used to love. This is due to the changes that cause pregnancy cravings in the first place, and the evolutionary origins of this chaotic pregnancy symptom.

What Causes Pregnancy Cravings?

There isn't quite a consensus in the medical community, but several theories have become popular. These center on changes to a pregnant woman's nutritional needs, hormones, senses, comfort, and even biological need to protect.

- Nutritional needs: The most obvious answer is that pregnant women simply need more nutrition to help the baby grow. Oftentimes pregnancy cravings will be for foods rich in necessary prenatal nutrients, like iron. One example of this is the common craving for ice cream, which is filled with calcium.

- Hormones: We don't fully understand every facet of the hormonal changes that women go through, and researchers believe the cause of cravings can be found within these changes. Hormones can change how you taste and smell food, thereby changing what types of food you crave and why.
- Senses: These same changes affect many of the senses, and can make pregnant women more sensitive to the smells of certain foods. If a food has an overwhelming odor, like some cheeses, your spouse may avoid it at all costs. Foods with a pleasant smell, like many fruits, can have the exact opposite effect.
- Comfort: Pregnancy is uncomfortable, and we don't call them "comfort foods" for nothing. Foods we associate with family or childhood, take-out from a favorite restaurant, or even a delicious morsel of candy: these can all help trigger your spouse's brain to release those feel-good chemicals that can lower their stress levels.
- Biological Need: Certain food aversion may be out of a biological imperative to protect an unborn child. Some pregnant women have

reported feeling sick at the smell of alcohol or coffee, and even the smell of meat. This is due to the possibility that these substances could be harmful or contaminated, and hurt the child. This theory does not apply to everyone, as some women crave coffee and meat even more.

It's Okay To Indulge, But Don't Overdo It

Nutrition is the cornerstone to a healthy pregnancy, and your partner should eat as much as they need to help the baby's growth. Making sure they get enough folic acid, calcium, protein, and iron is essential. But a healthy relationship with food is also important, and certain foods can even be dangerous.

There are several foods to avoid during pregnancy. These include:

- Sushi
- Undercooked (Rare) meat
- Low-quality meat, like deli meat
- Soft cheeses

These foods can be contaminated with bacteria, and while consumption could be perfectly fine, it's not worth the risk.

You should also watch for abnormal cravings. While I've never personally seen these, there are very worrisome cravings some women have reported thinking about during pregnancy. These include:

- Dirt
- Clay
- Ashes
- Paint Chips
- Laundry Detergent
- Raw cooking materials like starch and flour

While not common, it's still best to talk with your partner and ask how they are feeling. These strange cravings can often be caused by an iron deficiency, and you should talk to your doctor about blood tests to assess your spouse's iron levels.

CONSIDERING A MIDWIFE

As you near the halfway point in the pregnancy, it may be time to start considering whether or not you will use a midwife. A midwife is a pregnancy professional, trained to help women during labor, delivery, and for a short period after the birth. They can work in your home, their home, birthing centers, and sometimes even hospitals.

There are several different varieties of midwife, each with their own level of expertise. These include:

- Lay Midwives: These are non-certified, non-licensed midwives who have either apprenticed under a professional, or received some form of informal training.
- Certified Professional Midwives: Also referred to as CPMs, these midwives have experience in a birthing clinic or professional training. They usually have facilitated childbirth outside of a hospital, and have likely passed a national exam. Some states do not permit CPMs to operate.
- Certified Midwives: These midwives have completed their bachelor's degree or higher in a health-related field, along with an accredited program in midwifery. They have also passed a national exam. Like CPMs, certain states do not allow certified midwives to practice.
- Certified Nurse-Midwives: Certified nurse-midwives are allowed to practice in all 50 states, and have the highest level of credentials. They are registered nurses who have graduated from accredited education programs in both nursing and midwifery. They are also required to pass a national exam.

The care a midwife can provide covers many different facets of the pregnancy. Depending on their level of certification, midwives can:

- Administer prenatal exams and order tests
- Assist with preconception care and family planning
- Monitor the psychological and physical health of the mother
- Provide advice on exercise, medication, diet, and other ways to stay healthy
- Help you and your spouse make birthing plans
- Provide emotional and practical labor support
- Answer any questions you or your partner have about pregnancy, childbirth, and infant care
- Assist in admitting and discharging your spouse from the hospital
- Make necessary referrals to doctors
- Deliver your child

Using a midwife doesn't necessarily mean you won't need medical intervention, and they can often be a valuable resource in spotting complications early. We used a midwife for our second pregnancy, and it may have saved Leah's life.

For our first child, Alan, we decided on a home birth. We decided to use a midwife, and we interviewed several candidates and went with a person we trusted. As the due date came closer, our midwife noticed something that concerned her. She said due to the shape of Leah's hip bones, she believed there could be complications during the birth. Because of her advice, we decided to have Alan in a hospital. Thank god we did, because Leah needed her hip bones broken so Alan could be born. If we had stayed at home, or not had the advice of a trusted professional, I could have lost my wife and son.

Now that's just one person's story. Of course, not everyone can afford a midwife, and an at home birth isn't recommended for all pregnancies. You should discuss with your doctor whether your partner has the right health profile for an at-home or midwife-facilitated birth. More complicated birthing situations, like someone having twins, are an example of a situation where an at-hospital birth is usually required.

WHAT IS HAPPENING TO THE BABY DURING THE FOURTH MONTH?

By the end of this month your baby will be about 6 inches long and weigh nearly 4 ounces. They will start to develop their facial features, and begin to flex and clasp their hands, arms, and legs. It's also possible to see the baby's sex on an ultrasound, so the time will come to decide whether to see the gender early. Your baby will begin to produce their own estrogen and testosterone. More movement will also be happening, as your baby makes the most of the space in the amniotic sac. The baby will drink the fluid from this sac as well, and use it's kidneys to begin producing urine.

While the baby will be moving, we aren't quite at the stage where you'll feel "kicks". Later, once we get closer to month six and seven, you'll start to track these kicks to establish a pattern. At this point, there won't be much of a pattern to your baby's movement, but it's still exciting! Make sure your spouse appreciates these small movements while they can, because once the baby does start kicking it can aggravate certain pregnancy symptoms.

Between 16 and 18 weeks of pregnancy, your baby will be able to hear sounds from outside of the womb. This means you can talk to, and even play music to, your baby! Studies have shown that music can help develop areas of a baby's brain that assist language acquisition and future reading skills. You can also talk to or read to your unborn child; ultrasounds have shown babies reacting to their parent's voices.

FROM LEMON TO MANGO

As the second trimester continues, there will be more decisions to make concerning labor, birth, and what to do after leaving the hospital. Your baby will continue to grow at a healthy pace, with many features becoming more and more defined. Your partner will also need more help as the baby becomes more and more of a load. Let's take a look at what you can expect in month five.

LITTLE MANGO

"I'm your father, it is my job to protect you. It's a job I refuse to quit, and at which I can't afford to fail."

- James Avery, as Philip Banks on The Fresh Prince of Bel-Air

VOCABULARY FOR MONTH FIVE:

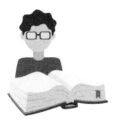

re·lax·in hor·mone	ep·som salts
/rə'laksiN 'hɔːməʊn/	/ˌepsəm 'sôlts/
*noun*MEDICINE Relaxin is a hormone produced by the ovary and the placenta with important effects in the female reproductive system and during pregnancy.	*noun*MEDICINE Epsom salts are crystals of hydrated magnesium sulfate used as a purgative or for other medicinal use.

ver·nix	la·nu·go
/'vərniks/	/lə'n(y)o͞oˌgō/
*noun*BIOLOGY noun: **vernix caseosa** The vernix is a greasy deposit covering the skin of a baby at birth.	*noun*BIOLOGY Lanugo is the fine, soft hair, especially that which covers the body and limbs of a human fetus or newborn.

mon·o·un·sat·u·rat·ed fats	round lig·a·ment pain
/ˌmänō ən saCHə ˌrādəd fāds/	/raʊnd-'lɪɡəmənt peɪn/
*adjective*CHEMISTRY Monounsaturated fats are an organic compound, specifically a fat, saturated except for one multiple bond.	*noun*MEDICINE Round ligament pain is a sharp pain or jabbing feeling often felt in the lower belly or groin area on one or both sides. It is one of the most common complaints during pregnancy and is considered a normal part of pregnancy. It is most often felt during the second trimester.

quick·en·ing	con·trac·tion
/'kwikəning/	/kən'trakSH(ə)n/
*noun*MEDICINE Quickening is defined as the first movements of the fetus felt in utero. It occurs from the eighteenth to the twentieth week of pregnancy. Movements have been felt as early as the tenth week and in rare cases are not felt during the entire pregnancy.	*noun*MEDICINE A shortening of the uterine muscles occurring at intervals before and during childbirth.

THE FIFTH MONTH

You've crested the hill and passed the halfway point in the pregnancy. At this point, many of the tasks you've undertaken to help your spouse will become second nature. Your home is slowly becoming an environment more conducive to a newborn, and you and your partner are likely becoming very excited. Those obnoxious pregnancy symptoms are beginning to subside, and you are both likely enjoying much less stress than you were in the first trimester. From here on out, the new symptoms that appear will be few. There are three primary additions in this fifth month: **swollen feet**, **lower back pain**, and an interesting phenomenon known as **Braxton Hicks contractions**.

Swollen Feet

As the months proceed, your partner may notice their feet swelling up. This can be a frustrating and painful symptom, but is a natural and explainable part of pregnancy. Several pregnancy-related factors contribute to giving your spouse swollen feet.

- Relaxin Hormone: Relaxin is a pregnancy hormone released by the ovaries and the placenta surrounding the baby. It works to promote implantation early in pregnancy, and in the second trimester it inhibits contractions in the uterine walls to prevent premature childbirth. Relaxin can also regulate the renal and cardiovascular systems to help mother's adapt to the increased oxygen and nutrient demand of the baby, and process the fetal waste products.

A side effect of this hormone's natural processes is also believed to be foot swelling. By relaxing the ligaments and stretching the tendons, the hormones will cause your partner's feet to flatten and increase in length.

- Fluid Retention: Increased water intake combined with the body's natural pregnancy mechanisms will cause women to retain fluid. This retention often affects the feet, and can be the root cause of the swelling.
- Weight Gain: The weight gained during pregnancy can also be a contributing factor to foot swelling. This is often why swelling becomes more pronounced the further into the pregnancy your partner gets; the weight of the fetus and uterus in the second and third trimester puts extra pressure on the feet and legs. This pressure usually causes the feet to swell.

Here are a couple of solutions you can use to help your partner relieve the swelling.

- Drink more water: While drinking too much water can contribute to feet swelling, dehydration can be just as problematic. It may not seem very logical, but getting the right amount of fluids helps reduce swelling. When you are dehydrated, your body does everything it can to preserve the fluids it has. By drinking more water, your body will stop retaining water and the swelling is likely to go down.

- Compression socks: Increased pressure to the legs can help maintain proper blood flow, reducing swelling and the associated discomfort. Compression socks are designed to apply this pressure slowly over time, and can be purchased online or in most pharmacies.

- Epsom salt bath: Magnesium sulfate, also known as Epsom salt, is a natural medicine that can help relieve swelling, inflammation, and muscle pain. It accomplishes by drawing out toxins and relaxing the muscles. When buying epsom salt, make sure it is an FDA approved brand marked with a "USP" label.

- Elevate your feet: Putting the feet up higher can help draw away blood and fluids, and slowly reduce painful swelling. Prop your partner's feet up on pillows or cushions several times a day for about 20 minutes at a time. If you can, help your partner avoid standing for too long while their feet are swollen. Get them to take breaks to elevate their feet at regular intervals until the swelling has subsided.

- Light exercise: Too much rest can be detrimental as well. Your partner should move a bit once every hour, whether that is a small walk, a couple of stretches, or standing up for a couple of minutes. Try to find a healthy balance between rest and light exercise, and the swelling should fade away.

Lower Back Pain

As the baby belly gets bigger, it begins to shift your spouse's center of gravity. This will cause her lower back to strain, and it will force supportive muscles to work harder than usual. Luckily, there are several remedies, including stretches you can do to strengthen lower back muscles.

- Backwards Stretch: Your partner should get on their hands and knees, keeping their hands beneath their shoulders and their arms straight out in front of them. Then, they'll curl back towards their heels as far as they can (without straining their knees.) Keeping their arms extended, your partner should tuck their head towards their knees, holding for several seconds then returning to their starting position. Repeat this 10 times, or as many times as is comfortable.

- Fitness Ball Stretch: If you have a fitness ball, or can easily purchase one, this stretch can help the pelvis and thighs along with the lower back. Similar to the backwards stretch, your partner will be on their knees with their hands straight out in front of them. Placing their hands on the exercise ball, they'll slowly curl backward towards their heels. Holding for several seconds, your partner will then return to their starting position. Repeat as many times as is comfortable.

- Pelvic Tilt: From a standing position, your partner should place their back against a wall with their feet shoulder-width apart. Pushing the small of their back against the wall, they will hold for several seconds before returning to their starting position. Repeat up to 10 times.

- Fitness Ball Pelvic Stretch: Have your partner sit on the floor with their back against the fitness ball, arms on their hips and feet on the floor. Then they will push their lower back upwards, and hold for several seconds. Return to the starting position and repeat up to 10 times.

- Torso Rotation: A good stretch for the upper back and torso, this stretch begins by sitting on the floor with legs crossed. Your partner will then hold their right foot with their left hand, and move their left hand slowly behind you. Open your upper body slowly to the right, and hold for several seconds before returning to the starting position. Perform 10 repetitions before switching to the other side.

Stretches are a great preventative measure, but sometimes there just isn't time. If your partner is experiencing lower-back pain and needs immediate relief, there are several temporary remedies you can try.

- Ice and Heat: Topical application of hot packs or ice packs is a great way to relieve back pain, but there is a certain procedure you should follow. Apply the ice packs first, then heat after. The cold will reduce any swelling, constrict the blood vessels to decrease inflammation, and numb the area to pain. Once any inflammatory symptoms have gone away, you can use a hot pack. This helps the muscles move, increasing the flexibility of soft tissues, and gets blood circulating so nutrients can repair those injured tissues.
- Medicated Creams: Topical painkillers, also known as analgesics, are applied to the top layer of skin wherever someone feels aches or

pains. These can come in the forms of creams, balms, or sprays, and there are various brands for different types of injuries. Make sure to check with your doctor before using any medications, as some creams will come with painkillers the baby may not react well to.

- Prop a pillow: An oldie but a goodie, simply prop a pillow or cushion under your partner's knees and ankles. This takes pressure off of the spine and lower back, and can help relieve pain and swelling.

Braxton Hicks Contractions

Braxton Hicks contractions can be a surprising and sometimes anxiety-inducing pregnancy symptom. You and your spouse will likely have similar questions I had when my wife experienced these "fake" contractions, so I've listed 5 I asked my doctor about.

1. What's the purpose of Braxton Hicks contractions?

Braxton Hicks contractions are basically a body's way of "practicing" for labor. They tone the uterine muscles, and get the cervix ready for the process of birth.

2. What do these contractions feel like?

Some women don't feel these contractions at all, but the ones that do have them report it as an abdominal tightness similar to a mild cramp. They usually don't last longer than 30 seconds, and are uncomfortable but rarely painful.

3. How can I make these contractions easier for my wife?

If the contractions are causing your partner any pain, which gets more common the closer you get to the due date, there are a few things you can do. Changing position can help, whether that is getting out of bed to take a short walk or sitting down and taking a rest. Whatever position she started in, try to change that and engage a different set of muscles. A light massage or warm bath can also be helpful. Deep breathing is a good stress reliever, and can help relax the muscles.

4. How can you tell the difference between these contractions and actual contractions?

Fortunately there are several very distinct differences between Braxton Hicks contractions from labor contractions. The duration is a good indicator: labor contractions will last between 30 and 70 seconds, while Braxton Hicks contractions will last less than 30 seconds. While you're timing the contractions, watch for a distinct pattern. If the contractions appear to get progressively stronger, that may indicate they are labor-induced. Braxton Hicks are irregular, and will often stop if your spouse changes her position or activity.

5. Okay, what should I do if I can't tell the difference?

If you have any doubt, contact your healthcare provider. They will be understanding, pregnancy is full of false alarms. Every woman is different, and premature births do occur. If you end up at a hospital by mistake, it's understandable to be embarrassed. Hospital staff are professionals, and will not judge you for making a small misstep. If anything, you can use a false alarm as a sort of practice run for the *real* thing.

BABYMOON

You and your partner have been working hard over the past 5 months, and you've passed the halfway point. While it isn't always possible, now would be a great time to celebrate with a Babymoon! A babymoon is like a honeymoon, but instead of happening after the wedding it happens before the birth. You'll probably be way too busy once the baby is born, so now would be a great time to enjoy a bit of alone time with your partner.

Having a babymoon before your first child is especially important, because this truly will be the end of an era. You and your partner have likely spent a long time together as a 2 person unit, and that's about to change forever. Taking one last trip for the two of you can be a romantic bonding experience you'll treasure for years to come.

For our trip, I knew Leah had always wanted to see the beautiful scenery of Banff National Park in Canada. So as a surprise, I booked a room at a little lodge and told her to take a week off of work. The look on her face when she saw the first "Banff National Park" road sign was priceless! We ended up having the cozy lodge to ourselves, spending the nights sipping hot cocoa by the fireplace and eating her favorite pregnancy craving combo: marbled cheddar cheese and saltine crackers. During the day, we wandered the town of Banff and walked the trails that wove through the mountains, lakes and forests. One of my favorite days ended with us finding this tiny overlook near Moraine Lake and taking a photo at sunrise. That photo still sits above our fireplace, and is a lovely reminder of such a special time in our lives.

Why Is The Second Trimester A Good Time For Travel?

The second trimester is ideal for a vacation as it's usually when pregnancy symptoms are at their lightest. The morning sickness has subsided, the baby bump isn't too big yet, and your partner's hormones have slowed down their constant barrage. There's just too much nausea and other problems during the first trimester, and it's usually a bit risky to travel during the third trimester, so the second is the best choice.

Talk to your partner about their dream destinations, and plan a "mock" extravagant trip just for fun. Pick everything you could possibly want to do, then start to decide what parts of the trip are absolutely essential. This is a good way to make a vacation fit your budget, and make sure you don't break the bank. For example, some people have a destination in mind, but don't really care about high-class accommodations. Hundreds can be saved on a trip by finding smaller and cozier sleeping arrangements instead of 5 star luxury hotels.

Talk to your doctor as well, and they'll let you know whether your pregnancy is low-risk enough to travel. You'll also want to check ahead of time what the medical services are like in the country you intend to travel to. Certain places also have higher risk of disease; Brazil, Honduras and Haiti, for example, have a large presence of malaria. Have fun, but be safe!

ANNOUNCING THE PREGNANCY

By month 5, you are well into the safe zone for telling friends and family. As the baby bump becomes more prominent, the subject will likely come up one way or another. You can have a large celebration, or let them know in passing conversation; how you let your loved ones know about the pregnancy is up to you.

Some couples choose to do a pregnancy announce-ment, which may be a fun way for you and your partner to bond. This can be something like a Christmas card, where you let people know you have a child on the way. There are custom card-making services that will let you choose the layout of this card, then you just send it in the mail.

If you decided to find out the gender, and want to reveal it to your friends and family, you could have a gender reveal party. Gender reveals are filled with fun events, food, and games centered around the reveal itself. The reveal usually involves showing the color blue if the baby is a boy, and the color pink if the baby is a girl. Just like a pregnancy announcement, you can tailor this event to you and your partner's personality. Have fun with it!

On a more work-related note, you will likely need to let your work know that you have a child on the way. This is especially important for your partner, who will have to go on maternity leave. They will likely need to to discuss with their boss about the proper protocols, and it doesn't hurt to get this figured out well ahead of time.

WHAT IS HAPPENING TO THE BABY DURING THE FIFTH MONTH?

At this stage, your baby will be around 5 inches long and weigh nearly 5 ounces at the beginning of the month. By the end, they could be as big as 10 inches, and weigh up to 1 pound. The baby will also begin to develop reflexes, like its throat muscles learning how to swallow. They'll also learn how to suck and latch onto things, and may even suck their thumb in-utero. Tooth buds will continue to develop, and the fingers and toes will become much more defined. The baby's skin will be bright pink at this point, but transparent and covered with a layer of soft, downy hair.

Your partner will notice a higher level of quickening this month, with increased movement, kicks, and flips.

These will likely begin to come at regular intervals, as your baby is starting to sleep and wake based on environmental events and noises. Your baby will also begin to produce vernix, a slick skin-protective coating inside the amniotic sac. This coating will be present when the baby is born, and cover their entire body. Lanugo will also begin to be produced, a fine soft layer of hair that holds the vernix into place. Unlike the vernix, Much of the lanugo will disappear before birth, though some will be present on small parts of the baby's skin.

FROM MANGO TO CAULIFLOWER

As you near the end of the second trimester, you may feel that stress slowly returning. The birth is getting closer, and you'll need a solid plan before that day comes. You'll also want to start considering childcare options, thinking of a baby name, and thinking of future fun events like a baby shower. Let's take a look at what you can expect in month six.

7

LITTLE CAULIFLOWER

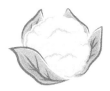

"Look, if it was up to me, you wouldn't have to sleep at all, you wouldn't have to go to school, I wouldn't have to go to work and we could just spend all our time together. And there's nothing I'd rather do."

- William Russ, as Alan Matthews on Boy Meets World

VOCABULARY FOR MONTH SIX:

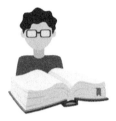

sur·fac·tant

/sər'faktənt/

*noun*ANATOMY

A surfactant is a substance which tends to reduce the surface tension of a liquid in which it is dissolved. In pregnancy, a surfactant makes it possible for babies to breathe in air after delivery.

ma·ter·ni·ty

/mə'tərnədē/

MEDICINE*noun*

Maternity refers to the period during pregnancy and shortly after childbirth.

al·ve·o·lus

/al'vēələs/

*noun*ANATOMY

plural noun: **alveoli**

Alveolus are any of the many tiny air sacs of the lungs which allow for rapid gaseous exchange.

li·ne·a ni·gra

/li·nee·uh nee·gruh/

*noun*ANATOMY

Linea nigra is a physiological form of hyperpigmentation commonly seen in the first trimester of pregnancy. It is a dark vertical line that runs down the middle of the abdomen and it can be one of the earliest indicators of pregnancy. It is also known as the 'pregnancy line'.

pre·term birth	hot flash
/prē tərm/ /bərTH/	/haat flasch/
MEDICINE*adjective* A preterm birth is when a child is born after a pregnancy significantly shorter than normal, especially after no more than 37 weeks of pregnancy.	(NORTH AMERICAN) *Noun* plural noun: **hot flashes** A hot flash is a sudden feeling of feverish heat, typically as a symptom of the menopause.

tach·y·car·di·a	nan·ny
/ˌtakəˈkärdēə/	/ˈnanē/
MEDICINE*noun* Tachycardia is an abnormally rapid or fast heart rate.	*noun* A nanny is a person, typically a woman, employed to care for a child in its own home.

THE SIXTH MONTH

As you enter the final month of the second trimester, you'll start to notice just how *quickly* time is moving. With all the excitement, doctors appointments, and planning, the months will begin to move more and more quickly. Try to take a couple of minutes every day, whether alone or with your partner, for quiet reflection. Now is a great time to go back over your journal, and see just how different your emotions are now than when you started. You'll be happy to see that many of those initial fears and concerns have been answered or abated; by this time, you'll hopefully have had ample time with medical professionals or other pregnancy experts, and provided them with every question you can think of. If you haven't, don't worry! You still have a couple of months.

Make sure to write down any question you can think of, even if you worry they may be "dumb questions." The truth is, there are no dumb questions; healthcare providers, more often than not, are happy when people want to to take a more active part in their partner's pregnancy. Asking questions means you care, and that empathetic quality will serve you well into fatherhood and beyond.

Now, let's talk about month six symptoms. As with last month, you'll really be dealing with much of the same: dizziness and back pain being two of the main culprits. The back pain will likely increase until the end of the pregnancy due to the rapid growth of the baby; the heavier your child gets, the more they will pull your partner forward and strain their back. Make sure to review the back pain tips and exercises in the previous chapter for ways to relieve your partner's back pain.

As for new symptoms, there are a couple of things that may pop-up. The most important affliction that will begin to rear its head in the sixth month is a little known pregnancy symptom: **hot flashes**.

Hot Flashes

Hot flashes are a symptom often associated with menopause, or the hormonal decline woman experience in their late 40's and 50's. As levels of estrogen and progesterone decline and production in the ovaries slows down, symptoms like hot flashes mark the end of the body's ability to reproduce. But why then would this symptom of the reproductive shutdown happen in a person who is actively reproducing?

The mechanism of action that causes hot flashes is the same in both women experiencing menopause and pregnancy. During pregnancy, sudden changes in estrogen and progesterone occur to help the baby develop; these changes mirror those that occur during menopause, so the body reacts in a similar way. Hot flashes are further exacerbated by the large calorie burning that happens during pregnancy, which can generate more heat than normal.

Hot flashes are usually present as an increase in perceived body temperature. Your partner may become uncomfortable and sweaty as they feel like every room they enter is a sauna. There are several ways you can help them deal with this symptom, including:

- <u>Hydration</u>: Seemingly the cure for all pregnancy related problems, proper hydration can drastically reduce the discomfort associated with hot flashes. This doesn't necessarily have to be glass after glass of boring old water either; when Leah was experiencing hot flashes, she happened to also be going through an endless craving for watermelon. So I thought, why not kill two birds with one stone? I found a sugar-free brand of watermelon popsicles that helped quench her thirst, cool her down, and satisfy her watermelon craving. Ask your partner what their favorite popsicle flavor is, and have a package ready for when they start to sweat.

- <u>Cold Air</u>: While you don't want to freeze your spouse completely, a fan near an open window can help relieve their hot flash symptoms. If they feel up to it, taking a seat outside when the temperatures are cooler, this can be a huge help as well. The fresh air combined with the cold can be refreshing, and help rid them of that uncomfortable heat.

- <u>Avoid Triggers</u>: Whether environmental or food-based, there are certain triggers for hot flashes you'll want to avoid if possible. Hot weather is a more obvious one; it's much easier to raise a temperature that's already being assisted by the sun. Stress is another environmental trigger, and if your partner begins to feel stressed out they may start to feel feverish. Caffeine can aggravate hot flashes as well, by raising your partner's heart rate and increasing their metabolic rate. Lastly, and this one is unfortunate for pregnancy craving sufferers, sugar has been known to trigger hot flashes as well. It may be a tough conversation, but talk to your partner about abstaining from the sweets if the sweats begin to bother them.

- Loose-fitting Clothing: The sixth month is a good time to purchase looser-fitting clothing for several reasons, but they are especially good for relieving hot flashes. Loose or flowy clothing allows the material to breath, so more cool air can circulate around the body. Tight-clothing can also increase stress, and may feel restrictive as the heat begins to bother your partner.

BUYING MATERNITY CLOTHES

Speaking of clothes, the beginning of the sixth month is a great time to get some comfortable pregnancy clothes. While your partner has likely found some looser-fitting clothing items to wear, the baby bump will become much bigger in the third trimester. But this doesn't have to be purely for utility; your partner should feel they can express themselves, especially if fashion is an important part of their individual identity.

Research highly-reputable maternity stores in your area and make a day of it. Depending on what months of the year the third trimester will take place, make sure to help them pick out the clothes they'll need. If it's summer, that means loose fitting and flowy clothes that will let them keep cool; if it's winter, they'll want large but warm clothing to keep them from getting chilly.

One of the most popular pieces of maternity clothing are dresses; whether it's simply an oversized dress, a slip, or wrap, these are easy to put on and don't put any undue pressure on the baby bump. This clothing doesn't need to go to waste after the baby is born either; oversized dresses make good nightwear, or you could donate the clothing to a local organization. You could also see if any of your friends are planning to have a baby, and see if they would like to use the same maternity clothing.

BIRTH PLAN

With three months left to go, it's time to lock down a birth plan. A birth plan is a document that you and your partner will craft concerning what procedures you would like to follow during labor and delivery. You will show this plan to your midwife or medical team; it will usually cover things like how your partner would like to manage their pain, what should happen to the baby they're born with, and your plans for immediate post-partum care.

Before making your plan, you should decide what type of birth your partner is trying to have. If you plan to do an at-home birth or use a midwife, you'll want to make sure you have every piece of equipment prepared and ready. A midwife can help you craft a plan even if you decide to go to a hospital, so it's in your best interest to seek one out.

If you do decide to go to a hospital, the first thing you should do is inspect the facility. Take a short tour, and ask questions about what the delivery ward is equipped with. Do they have a birthing tub, or is it the more traditional stirrups and hospital bed set up? What pain management plans do they offer? Do they only do epidurals, or will they also have alternative pain medications like nitrous oxide. How many people can be in the delivery room during labor? This is a good question to ask if you have a midwife, because they may only allow family members in the delivery rooms.

Make part of your plan greeting the staff when you arrive. Unless the delivery is planned and induced at a specific time, you will likely be dealing with whoever is on call when your wife goes into labor. This will be who delivers your baby. If you can, briefly run them through your birth plan so they know what your ideal situation would entail. Introduce them to any support person you happen to bring, whether it be your midwife or a relative. At the same time, be understanding; medical staff usually know what's best, but will still try to do everything they can to accommodate you.

Let the staff know your partner's personal preferences as well. Anything that may make them uncomfortable, whether that is a male doctor, brightly lit room, or medical interns bumbling around, you can let them know. This will be a difficult time for your partner, and anything you can do to reduce their stress will help the delivery go smoother.

Once the baby is born, you should have a plan for what you would like to happen. If you have decided to have your baby circumcised, you need to decide whether that will happen at the hospital or in a separate location. Your partner also may want to keep the baby near her immediately after delivery, and that should be brought up to the staff as well.

One thing to remember with all good plans is that things go awry; but again, no need to panic! These healthcare professionals have likely seen every possible scenario, and will have contingency procedures for any eventuality. Your birth plan will serve as a set of guidelines for them to work along, but they will be more than equipped to handle any issue that should arise.

CHILDCARE OPTIONS

As the third trimester begins, it's time to look forward to the future. Who will care for your child when you return to work? While your partner will likely get some maternity leave, you will probably not get the same time off. The postpartum period can be difficult for mothers, and caring for the baby alone could be overwhelming. Hiring a support staff member, like a maid or nanny, can help reduce some of the workload new moms experience. It isn't fair to expect your partner to keep the entire house clean, take care of the newborn, and work on her pregnancy recovery. While you should be using any extra time you have to help out, there may not be enough hours in the day.

Hiring a nanny may be a necessity, but there are several steps you should take beforehand. Here are eight steps you can take to make sure you get the best possible care for your child:

1. *Discuss Preferences:* You and your partner should discuss what you are both looking for in a nanny, and assemble a list of preferences. Make sure to take into account not only the needs of your baby, but your spouse as well. Part of this conversation are the duties you would expect of a nanny. Will this person be helping with housework? Assistance with activities like laundry, cooking, and vacuuming can give your partner more time to rest and focus on your child. Visitors will have another preference to discuss. Can the nanny invite someone over, or take the child on play dates? Socialization is good for children, but taking your child outside of the home may make you uncomfortable. Restricting your child's access to electronics may be another duty you expect from a nanny. If you don't want your child sitting in front of a tv or ipad all day, you'll need to let your nanny know. Make sure to have all of this ready to go before you begin your first interview.

2. *Don't Start Your Search Late:* If you are starting your search for a nanny before the baby is born, that's good. While starting too early, like the first trimester, is unnecessary, you don't want to wait until the baby has already been delivered. Finding a nanny last minute can lead

you to compromising and choosing a subpar candidate. You want to find your person ahead of time to avoid undue stress.

3. *Look For Experience:* For any support staff you hire, you'll want someone with years of experience dealing with children. You also may need to look for someone who specializes in your specific child care situation; if you have twins, or a child with a developmental disorder, you'll need to look for nannies who have dealt with that specific scenario.

4. *Interview Multiple Candidates:* Part of finding the right person is interviewing multiple people before hiring someone. It may be difficult to find the time to interview multiple nannies in person; thankfully, modern technology has your back. Organize video or phone calls and find time to talk to a decent sized group of candidates. Don't rush this process; you want to find someone you can trust in your home when you are away, and who will facilitate the healthy growth of your child. A calm, kind demeanor from a candidate is a plus!

5. *Identify Red Flags:* As with any situation, you'll want to look for red flags that someone may not be a good fit for your family. You should not feel bad for filtering out candidates that

make you uncomfortable; trust your gut, and make the decisions you need to make when it comes to your family's safety. If a nanny seems like they may be untrustworthy, or hiding something that could bring your family harm, move on to another candidate.

6. *Check References:* One way to determine whether a person is free of red flags and has the right experience is references. Any nanny you consider should have a list of personal and professional references, people you can call to determine how well this person will perform their duties. Make sure to ask questions like "Would you hire this person again?", "What issues did you experience during this person's employment?", and "What are some examples of times this person went above and beyond to help you?".

7. *Clearly Lay Out Pay Expectations:* Once you've gotten a bit further into the interview process, discuss compensation. Have a set price beforehand, and make sure the nanny is okay with your budget. Discuss what days off the person would prefer, and whether or not they would like vacation time. Talk about how often payments will happen, and whether they'll be paid hourly or on a flat rate. Make sure to

properly document all of these agreements, so there is less chance of a dispute in the future.

8. *Let The Nanny Shadow You:* If you land on someone you think would be a good fit, have them shadow you for the first couple of days. Let them see how you take care of your baby, so they can emulate your behavior. Walk them through how you handle changing diapers, crying, playtime, and putting the baby to sleep. Once you've shown them, watch them perform these tasks so you can make sure they are done correctly.

WHAT'S HAPPENING TO THE BABY DURING THE SIXTH MONTH?

There isn't a huge amount of new developments between the fifth and sixth month, but your child will change in several important ways. By the sixth month, your baby will weigh more than a pound and be almost one whole foot long. This is the month the baby really starts moving, and will usually react to any loud noises or speech.

The baby's sense of hearing is fully developed. Their skin is reddish in color, and spider webbing vein systems can be seen below their translucent skin. Their eyes will begin to move rapidly behind their closed eyelids, and their lungs are completely formed (though not yet fully-functional). A baby will also have developed their sucking reflex almost completely, and could even be seen sucking its thumb via ultrasound.

FROM CAULIFLOWER TO BUTTERNUT SQUASH

The second trimester is coming to a close, and you are entering the final stretch of the pregnancy. Things may start to ramp back up here, but there's no need to worry. As long as you've taken the time to prepare yourself and help your partner, you should have no trouble navigating the slight turbulence ahead. The time is coming to shift your focus from the pregnancy itself to the period of time immediately after, when your baby is a newborn. Let's take a look at what you should start to consider, and what you can expect, in the seventh month.

8

LITTLE BUTTERNUT SQUASH

"Steven, I've come to think of you as a son. So I want to give you some honest, heartfelt advice."

- Kurt Woodman, as Red Forman on That 70's Show

VOCABULARY FOR MONTH SEVEN:

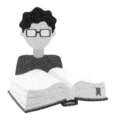

child care

/ˈCHīld ˌker/

noun

Childcare is defined as the action or skill of looking after children.

rho·gam

/ˈRow gm/

noun

RhoGAM, or RhO(D) immune globulin, is an injectable drug that is used to protect an Rh+ fetus from antibodies in an Rh- mother's blood and to prevent Rh allergy in the mother.

stretch marks

/ˈstreCH ˌmärks/

noun

Irregular lines or streaks on the skin where it has been stretched or distended, especially due to pregnancy or obesity.

nerv·ous sys·tem

/ˈnərvəs ˌsistəm/

noun

The network of nerve cells and fibers which transmits nerve impulses between parts of the body.

e·pi·si·ot·o·my

/iˌpēzēˈädəmē/

noun

A surgical cut made at the opening of the vagina during childbirth, to aid a difficult delivery and prevent rupture of tissues.

mel·a·nin

/ˈmelənən/

noun

A dark brown to black pigment occurs in the hair, skin, and iris of the eye in people and animals. It is responsible for tanning of skin exposed to sunlight.

fi·ber	pel·vis
/ˈfībər/	/ˈpelvəs/
noun	*noun*
Dietary material containing substances such as cellulose, lignin, and pectin, that are resistant to the action of digestive enzymes.	The large bony structure near the base of the spine to which the hind limbs or legs are attached in humans and many other vertebrates.

THE SEVENTH MONTH

As we enter the third trimester, the due date starts to become a more powerful reality. In a few short months, you will be a dad; much like when you were first told, that excitement and fear may start to bubble up again. Stay cool, you've got this! Take some alone time during this month and put some energy into your hobbies. You've likely been neglecting some of your passions due to all the work you've been doing, and while preparing for the baby is essential, it's good to do something for yourself as well.

As for new symptoms, there are several that may begin to bother your partner during month seven. While familiar afflictions like fatigue and Braxton Hicks contractions will start to ramp up during this month, your spouse will also begin to feel three newer symptoms: **pelvic pain**, **sciatica**, and **constipation**.

Pelvic Pain

The ever increasing size of the baby, combined with an increase in pregnancy hormones, can often result in feelings of pelvic pain. As the baby gets bigger, the space inside your partner's body gets smaller. This puts pressure on the pelvis, and can strain the muscles. Pregnancy hormones like progesterone can aggravate the pelvis as well; progesterone loosens the joints connecting the sides of the pelvis to help prepare the body for labor and delivery.

While pelvic pain during pregnancy is perfectly normal and rarely indicative of deeper issues, you'll probably want to help your partner relieve their discomfort. There are several actions you can take to give your spouse relief, including:

- Water Exercises: Water buoyancy is a great way to take strain off of the joints, and water exercises can help work the pelvic area without causing further pain. Try to find an aqua aerobics class in your area, or help your spouse gently swim laps in the pool.
- Pelvic Stretches: A great way to accompany any exercises is a good stretching regimen. Pelvic stretches can help strengthen the pelvic floor, along with the hip, back, and stomach muscles.

- Rest: Your partner should acknowledge when they are feeling a bout of pelvic pain, and take the time to rest. Ignoring pain signals, especially when they become strong, can cause further strain. Communicate with your spouse, and ask them if they need a second to sit or lie down.
- Supportive Shoes: High-quality supportive shoes are a good way to relieve pain in the lower body, and can help make activities like walking rejuvenate your partner instead of hurting them.
- Ice: An old stand-by, ice, is a great way to reduce inflammation in any part of the body. Simply put an icepack or other cooling device onto your partner's pelvic joints for periods of about 15 minutes. Be careful not to leave these on too long, as they can damage the skin.

Sciatica

As your partner's uterus grows larger, pressure will be applied to different areas of her body. One area that acutely experiences this pressure is the sciatic nerve. When pressed, this nerve will cause a type of pain known as sciatica. Sciatica can be felt in the hips and lower back, and usually travels down one of the legs.

This pain can feel like a burning sensation, numbness, weakness, or even a sharp stabbing shock.

The good news is , sciatic pain will usually resolve on its own without intervention. But, you'll still want to help your partner feel better while sciatica is afflicting them. There are several ways to do this, including:

- Change Position: Whatever position your partner is in when the sciatica strikes, it's best to move to see if the pain will be relieved. If the pain hits while sitting, stand up; if you are standing, try lying down. Too much rest can weaken the muscles, and actually aggravate the sciatica. It's best to get light exercise in, if your partner is feeling up to it.
- Get Moving: Speaking of too much rest, movement is an effective way to relieve the pain of sciatica. As long as the pain isn't too severe, take a short walk with your partner if they are experiencing a flare-up. Moving around can adjust the pressure on the sciatic nerve and help relieve symptoms.
- Heat: While cold can also be helpful, a hotpack is a good way to reduce the feelings of pain associated with sciatica. Warm towels or heating pads are a good way to transfer heat to

the pelvic area, and can also be used on the lower back and hips.

Constipation

A combination of that pesky pregnancy hormone progesterone and the high levels of iron in prenatal vitamins can often slow down a person's digestion; this will cause their digestive system to become backed up. This is usually called constipation, and it can be a very uncomfortable situation to deal with. There are a couple of ways you can help your spouse, including:

- Hydration: Seemingly the cure to all problems, proper hydration can help revitalize the digestive system, causing clogged pathways to open up and allow waste to be eliminated. Water can also help soften the stool, making it much easier to pass.
- Fibrous Foods: Foods that are high in fiber are not only a great way to improve digestive help, but can eliminate the issues associated with constipation. Fiber helps stool soak up water, so it can solidify and easily leave the body.
- Prune Juice: Prune juice combines the hydration powers of water and the fiber-content of fibrous foods to drastically relieve the symptoms of

constipation. One of the best parts of prune juice is that it also comes with a sugar alcohol called sorbitol. Sorbitol helps further soften the stool to make bowel movements much easier.

• Prebiotic and Probiotic Supplements: Both prebiotics and probiotics aid in the development and maintenance of a healthy colony of bacteria and other microorganisms in the gut, which supports digestion. By supplying food and creating an environment in which good bacteria can thrive, these food components aid in the promotion of beneficial bacteria.

BABY CLOTHES

Now is the time to start thinking about what your little squash is going to be wearing in the first couple of months out of the womb. While infant clothes are essential, it's important you don't go overboard; many of these outfits will obviously be obsolete as the baby rapidly grows in their first year. There are several items you'll want to get for your child, usually ranging between two and eight pieces for each clothing type.

These types include:

- Onesies: Onesies are great for easily dressing your infant, and don't take too much struggle to get over their sensitive arms and legs. You'll want between four and eight onesies for your baby.
- Infant Gowns: Gowns are good for immediately after the baby is born, when you'll need to constantly clean the area where the umbilical cord was. It also provides easy diaper access so changing isn't such a hassle. You'll want between two and four infant gowns.
- Undershirts: These will go underneath whatever outwear your baby has, and likely snap under their crotch or over their shoulder. You'll want between four and eight undershirts.
- Pajamas: The baby's nightwear should be comfortable, but made of an easily-washable material in case of night-time accidents. You'll want between four and eight pajamas for your baby.
- Sweaters or Jackets: Especially important for the colder months, sweaters and jackets will usually button in the front to allow the baby to lie down. You'll want between one and three sweaters or jackets.

- Rompers: You don't necessarily need rompers for your baby, but they do make a cute outfit for going out and showing off to friends and family. If you do get rompers, you'll only need one or two.
- Hats: Keeping the sun out of your baby's eyes and off of their sensitive skin is important, and hats are a good way to keep your child's body in the shade. Again, a washable hat is preferred, as they are usually in the splash-zone for spit up. You'll want between three and five hats, with wide brims to block the sun.
- Mittens: Keeping your child's hands warm is important, and mittens are a good way to keep their little fingers nice and toasty. One pair of mittens is usually fine.
- Bunting Bag: A bunting bag is like a little sleeping bag for your baby, and is more important in snowy winter environments. One bunting bag should do fine.

There are several ways you can acquire your baby clothes: purchasing them on your own, finding hand-me-downs, or putting them in your baby registry. If you choose to purchase them on your own, remember that most of these clothing items will not be used in a couple of months to a year. Talk to your friends, or other parents in your baby groups, and see if they have any hand-me-downs from any past pregnancies. Leah and her mom go to an annual garage sale every year, so they were able to find a large amount of our baby's clothing at an affordable price. You can also put baby clothes in the registry for your baby shower (something we will talk about in the next chapter). This way, you'll receive a good amount of the outfits as gifts and save that money for other important baby items.

STAYING AT HOME

Something to consider as you get closer to the delivery is whether or not your partner will stay home to spend more time with the child. Now this is important: while you can help your partner make this decision, it is ultimately up to them. You can't ask your wife to sacrifice her current career any more than she can ask you to sacrifice yours. That being said, Leah and I had many discussions as the due date grew closer. She eventually decided she would stay home, and her mom was a big inspiration for that decision.

When Leah told her parents she was pregnant, they were overjoyed. They live close to our home, and her mom offered to help in any way she could. Leah's mother also chose to stay at home for her children, despite her husband promising they could make it work. It's possible it would have worked; many parents find a balance of childcare and career that creates a healthy environment for a child to grow up in. But Leah's mom wanted to spend as much time as possible with her children, and she said it was one of the best decisions she ever made. I've seen the photo albums, and it always warms my heart to see my wife as a child in front of movie theaters, in parks, and riding around in a shopping cart. Leah told me that getting off the bus everyday and having her mom there was incredibly special. Her mother took her everywhere, and it made their bond that much stronger in the future. Now she gets to create those same memories with our children.

All of that said, there is nothing wrong with not taking the more traditional route. If your partner's career is fulfilling, they should be able to experience that achievement. You may even want to consider staying home yourself. All options should be discussed when talking about childcare. Whatever you choose, just make sure you find as much time to spend with your child as possible. Those early years are so precious, and I've never regretted a single moment I spent with my children; only the moments that I missed.

WHAT IS HAPPENING TO THE BABY DURING THE SEVENTH MONTH?

During the seventh month, the baby's body is preparing itself to exit the womb. Many fascinating processes are occurring during this time, including the continued production of surfactant. As this substance builds up, it allows your baby's lungs to expand and contract as they will outside of the mother's body. Your baby will also begin to fully open and close their eyes, and sense environmental changes outside of the belly. You may notice that as your partner moves from a darker area to a brighter one, the baby may respond with a little kick or movement. This will also happen with sound, as the ears start to pick up on familiar vibrations like your partner's voice.

Melanin will also start to be produced during this month, a natural skin pigment that gives the baby's skin (and yours) its color. The baby will begin to lose the reddish-pink hue to their skin and start to look more like they will once they're born. Your child will also begin to gain a bit of weight and start to get that adorable "pudgy" look we often associate with newborns. Beyond being cute, the extra fat also serves the purpose of smoothing out the many wrinkles a baby has in utero.

FROM BUTTERNUT SQUASH TO PINEAPPLE

You are in the home stretch now, and the suspense may begin to mount for you and your partner. Nothing eases that tension like a nice date night, and it may be good to take your spouse out for a romantic meal before the baby bump becomes too burdensome. Take some time this month to absorb the silence of your home; while children are a joy, silence will be one commodity that you'll find in short supply during the first few years. As we move from the seventh month to the eighth, we'll be looking at the various ways you can prepare your home for the arrival of your child. Let's take a look at what you can expect in month eight.

9

LITTLE PINEAPPLE

"*Laughter's the best medicine, right? I'm keeping it loose, keeping it light.*"

- Ray Romano, as Ray Barone on Everybody Loves Raymond

VOCABULARY FOR MONTH EIGHT:

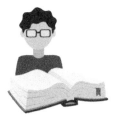

la·bor	CPR
/ˈlābər/	/ˌsēˌpēˈär/
noun	*noun*
The process of childbirth, especially the period from the start of uterine contractions to delivery.	Short for cardiopulmonary resuscitation.a medical procedure involving repeated compression of a patient's chest, performed in an attempt to restore the blood circulation and breathing of a person who has suffered cardiac arrest.

fon·ta·nel	var·i·cose
/ˌfäntnˈel/	/ˈverəˌkōs/
noun	*noun*
A space between the bones of the skull in an infant or fetus, where ossification is not complete and the sutures are not fully formed. The main one is between the frontal and parietal bones.	Affected by a condition causing the swelling and tortuous lengthening of veins, most often in the legs.

hem·or·rhoid	di·a·phragm
/ˈhem(ə)ˌroid/	/ˈdīəˌfram/
noun	*noun*
A swollen vein or group of veins in the region of the anus.	A dome-shaped muscular partition separating the thorax from the abdomen in mammals. It plays a major role in breathing, as its contraction increases the volume of the thorax and so inflates the lungs.

hy·po·thal·a·mus	ep·som salts
/ˌhīpəˈTHaləməs/	/ˌepsəm ˈsôlts/
noun	*noun*
A region of the forebrain below the thalamus which coordinates both the autonomic nervous system and the activity of the pituitary, controlling body temperature, thirst, hunger, and other homeostatic systems, and is involved in sleep and emotional activity.	Crystals of hydrated magnesium sulfate used as a purgative or for other medicinal use.

THE EIGHTH MONTH

With only two months left, you will begin to shift your focus away from the pregnancy itself and set your eyes towards the future. The eighth month will be spent preparing your home for the arrival of a new tiny roommate; unfortunately, this roommate will be very accident-prone, messy, and will rarely do their own dishes. This will also be a month for celebration, and is an excellent time to throw a baby shower.

As with every month, there will be new and persisting symptoms to help your partner work through. While she has likely adjusted to the fatigue and frequent urination, three new ailments will begin to bug her in the eighth month: **Shortness of breath, varicose veins,** and **hemorrhoids.**

Shortness of Breath

During the third trimester, your baby will be nearing the size it will be at birth. This means it is pushing your partner's uterus up against their diaphragm, and can move as far as 4 centimeters away from where it sat prepregnancy. This compresses the lunges, causing the anxiety-inducing feeling we know as "shortness of breath." This can make your spouse incredibly uncomfortable; reduced oxygen can make people hyperventilate and even pass out, which can be very dangerous for both the mother and child.

The first step to helping your partner overcome shortness of breath is to find a calming environment. Help them move to a spot free of noise and bright lights, and ask them to take a deep breath. As they do, explain to them what I said in the paragraph above; it's amazing what a logical explanation can do for stress-aggravated symptoms like shortness of breath. There are also several other solutions you can try, including:

- Pursed-lip Breathing: Pursed-lip breathing is a pacing technique that can help slow down the intake of air, making each breath deeper and far more effective. Pursing your lips can help you empty the lungs of dead air, taking in more fresh, oxygen-rich air. To perform pursed lip breathing, simply relax the neck and shoulder while slowly breathing in through your nose for two seconds. Then, purse your lips as though you are about to whistle, and gently breath out for four seconds.

- Back-supported Stand: While sitting down may seem like the most logical move and may be the best choice if your partner is feeling dizzy, a back-supported stand can also help relax and fill the airways. Have your partner stand against a wall with their feet shoulder-width apart and their hands on their thighs. Help them lean forward slightly, but not too far to crunch over their belly. This position gives them more space to fill up their chest and lungs.

- Using a Fan: A large part of shortness of breath is in the mind, and using a fan to blow cool air can help relieve the anxiety that often accompanies this symptom. The fan will not only help direct more air towards the mouth and lungs, but will help the sweating that can accompany a bout of breathlessness.

- Speak Calming Words: Calmly speaking to your wife while rubbing her shoulders, stomach, feet, etc. can encourage her to take deeper breaths. Oftentimes I would talk to Leah and ask her to tell me about good things. This would shift her focus to grateful topics and I would ask her to go in depth on what she was saying. We would also talk to our unborn baby together, telling them stories or even singing a lullaby.

Varicose Veins

We briefly covered skin and vein changes in chapter 5, but varicose veins can be a bit more troublesome than a simple cosmetic issue. If a vein becomes varicose, it will enlarge and push closer to the surface of the skin. These veins will usually be blue or purple in color, raised, and may be sore or itchy. They are most likely to appear on the legs due to the extra weight they have been tasked with carrying.

While more serious cases of varicose veins may require surgery, most of the time you just need to relieve the pain. This can be done by:

- Doing Leg Stretches: Stretching out the calves for several short periods every day can help significantly reduce the pain from varicose veins. A good way to do this is by flexing the feet while sitting, pushing the toes forward and backward to activate the calf muscles. Taking breaks from standing too long is also a good way to give your legs a break, and relieve the tension built up in the veins.
- Soaking In Cold Water: It may sound unpleasant, but cold water is a great way to reduce the pressure built up in varicose veins. The cold temperature of the water can cause the leg's blood vessels to shrink, which will reduce the pain signals shooting to the brain.
- Wearing The Right Clothes: Tight pants or high heeled shoes can often be pain triggers for those suffering from varicose veins. Wearing comfortable, loose-fitting clothes and shoes that don't restrict your feet can help blood flow more freely.

Hemorrhoids

The increased amount of blood present in a pregnant woman's body combined with a higher-rate of blood circulation can result in a painful symptom known as hemorrhoids. Much like varicose veins, hemorrhoids are veins that have pushed to the surface of the skin and can become irritated and itchy. Hemorrhoids appear near the rectal area, and result from the pressure caused by the uterus. This uterine pressure restricts the blood flow to and from the lower body and irritates the veins.

Hemorrhoids are likely to happen at some point in the pregnancy (most likely the third trimester); there is no real way to avoid them. There are several ways you can alleviate the more obnoxious symptoms of hemorrhoids, like:

- OTC Remedies: Over-the-counter, or OTC, is a class of medication that you can buy without a prescription. These medications range from medicated lotions, to painkillers and sanitizers. For hemorrhoids, you'll want to try witch hazel. Placing medicated witch hazel pads over the affected area can help reduce the swelling and pain. There are also medicated creams you can apply, though you'll want to talk to your doctor before using any medication during pregnancy.
- Avoid Sitting As Much As Possible: The pressure caused by sitting can further inflame the rectal veins, so avoiding sitting whenever your partner can is a good relief technique. Lying on their side or standing up is preferable,

and when they have to sit down (to rest, work, or anything else) make sure they take frequent breaks. Sitting on a comfortable pillow or hemorrhoid ring can also be helpful, as this takes pressure off of the affected area.

- Soaking in Warm Water: Not only is a nice hot bath relaxing, but it can also help reduce the size of hemorrhoids. A good way to increase the effectiveness of a warm water soak is epsom salt; epsom salt soothes the muscles, and can help relieve the pressure causing your partner's hemorrhoids.

7 TIPS TO THROWING A BABY SHOWER

While this is often done by family and friends, throwing a baby shower for your spouse can be a good way to give your partner some quality socialization and much-needed baby items. Setting up a shower isn't too difficult, and I actually helped plan baby showers for each of our children. Here are some easy guidelines you can follow to throw a great baby shower.

1. *Set-up a Baby Registry*: Before the party, make sure to set up a baby registry. A baby registry is a list of items you would like to receive as gifts; this can either be put on your invites, or exist within an online marketplace like Amazon. It may seem a bit awkward to ask for certain items, but believe me, people appreciate it. Instead of searching around for what gift to get, or risking getting something that won't be used, your guests will be able to rest easy knowing they got you a gift you'll love.

2. *Send Out Invitations*: It may seem obvious, but the first step to having any event is inviting the event's participants. Think about what guests your wife would like to see, and send them an invite via the mail, phone, or social media. The invite should have the time of the shower, date, location, and baby registry information.

3. *Decide On a Theme*: You don't necessarily need to have a theme, but a baby shower theme can help make planning the food and decorations a bit easier. For example, Leah is a big fan of the snow, so for her first shower we did a "Winter Wonderland" theme. Our son Alan chose the theme for the second shower...sort of. He was two, so he wanted the theme to be Monsters Inc. Whatever theme you choose, make sure it's

something your partner enjoys and is appropriate for your guests.

4. *Plan the Food*: Make sure to ask your guests what food allergies they have when you invite them, so you can more easily plan the menu. Keeping the dishes healthy is a good idea as well, and make sure they are all pregnancy friendly. That means no sushi, or cigars!

5. *Decorate*: Your decorations should keep in line with your theme, and generally relate to childbirth and the baby. There's no need to go crazy with decorations; a nice welcome sign, colorful flowers, and a few balloons can work perfectly well.

6. *Choose the Games*: Games are the foundation of a good baby shower and can be a lot of fun. They also help break the ice if your guests aren't all familiar with each other. These games or activities can really be anything; for example, you could paint one wall of the nursery together, adding little drawings and personal touches. Whatever you decide on, the activity should be something your partner can participate in easily.

7. *Consider Baby Shower Favors*: While certainly not required, giving out baby shower favors is a nice way to thank your guests for coming and

154 | NIGEL BOYD

giving gifts of their own. These can be small trinkets, nothing too fancy or expensive; a scented lotion, chocolates, and a small thank you card works great.

PREPARING YOUR HOME FOR THE BABY

While by now you've likely selected your child's room and furnished the space, there is still the matter of preparing your entire home for the arrival of a baby. It's difficult to understand, but your child will be crawling before you know it. You need to prep each space within your home to ensure it's safe for your child to enter unsupervised. It's impossible to keep eyes on your little ones 24 hours a day, so proper preparation is the best solution.

- General Changes: Each room will have specific actions that you need to complete, but there are some overarching changes for your house in general, like outlet cord coverings. Making sure that your home is equipped with a large first aid kit is important. You'll want cleaning wipes, antibiotic creams, baby aspirin, and bandages for small cuts and scrapes. It also wouldn't hurt for you to get certified in infant CPR as a precautionary measure.

- The Bathroom: The bathroom can be a dangerous place for a crawling infant, but there are ways to babyproof several key spots within your bathroom to make it safe. Make sure all medications are locked away or far out of the reach of a babies prying hands. Make sure to have locks on anything that could endanger your child: this includes the toilet seat, garbage can, and any cabinets they may try to get inside.
- The Kitchen: The kitchen can contain many objects that can injure your child, including sharp knives, stovetops, and cleaning supplies. You want to have covers for all stove knobs so they can't be turned on by your baby, and make sure to cook on burners that are outside of their reach. Never leave sharp objects out on the counter, and secure all the cabinets like you did in the bathroom. Unplugging appliances and storing them out of your child's way is also necessary, so your child does not operate any equipment while unattended.
- The Living Room: Make sure to cover all table corners and other sharp edges so your child does not bump or scratch themselves. You also want to move any electrical or window cords out of the way, as your baby can accidentally strangle themselves if you aren't careful. If your

living room has a fireplace, make sure to never leave your child near it when lit. Even if the fireplace has a glass screen, the heated surface can still injure your child if touched.

- Laundry Room: The most important step to securing your laundry room is to store detergents and other chemicals out of the way. We personally keep many cleaning supplies in our laundry room, but they are stored on a very high shelf. I also made sure that a baby could not crawl up to any higher points; be wary of step-like furniture that can offer your child a climbing route.

Your House May Differ

The layout of your home may be different, so the most important thing is to apply general safety precautions to each room. The big things to look out for are:

- Chords, ropes, and strings
- Chemicals or other poisonous materials
- Sharp, hot, or electrified objects
- Any way the baby can get up high

WHAT IS HAPPENING TO THE BABY DURING THE EIGHTH MONTH?

The eighth month is the beginning of a rapid increase in weight for the baby, hence the growing symptoms related to the pressure and uterine expansion. Your baby will be between 17 and 20 inches in length, and weigh anywhere from 5 to 7 pounds. Each week, the baby will gain half a pound, until reaching their final delivery weight.

The fine hair that covers your baby, called lanugo, will start to disappear in the eighth month. Your child will also become more active, and kicks will become a frequent occurrence. Your doctor will most likely recommend you count the number of movements that happen each day, as this can function as a way to check the health of the unborn child.

The baby's brain will grow as well this month, including increased development of the hypothalamus. This part of the brain will allow the baby to control its temperature, which they will need once they exit the safety of the womb. Your child's bones will also start to harden, but not the skull; that needs to be pliable to pass through the birth canal during delivery.

FROM PINEAPPLE TO WATERMELON

Here it is; we're moving into the final month. The ninth month involves final preparations for the baby's arrival, and then your experience at the hospital itself. It may sound scary, but babies are born every day; the medical professionals who will facilitate the delivery will know exactly what to do, and be there with you every step of the way. Let's take a look at what you can expect in month nine!

LITTLE WATERMELON

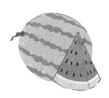

'Wow, I can't believe it, I wanted to make some kids that I could teach good and bad, right and wrong...and now I can! All I gotta do is be a good parent. Note to self: Good parents don't leave their kids home alone."

- Tom Kane, as the voice of Professor Utonium on The Powerpuff Girls

VOCABULARY FOR MONTH NINE:

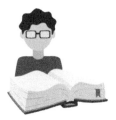

ce·sar·e·an sec·tion

/səˈzerēən/ /ˈsekSH(ə)n/

noun

A surgical procedure used to deliver a baby through incisions in the abdomen and uterus.

swad·dle

/ˈswädl/

verb

To wrap (someone, especially a baby) in garments or cloth.

for·mu·la

/ˈfôrmyələ/

noun

An infant's liquid food preparation based on cow's milk or soy protein, given as a substitute for breast milk.

de·liv·er·y

/dəˈliv(ə)rē/

noun

The process of giving birth.

af·ter·birth

/ˈaftərˌbərTH/

noun

The placenta and fetal membranes are discharged from the uterus after the birth of offspring.

breech

/brēCH/

adjective

Relating to or denoting presentation of a fetus in which the buttocks, rump, or legs are nearest the cervix and emerge first at birth.

THE NINTH MONTH

The time has arrived: the final month. You may get a bit of anxiety as the reality of momentous change sets in, but I encourage you to breathe. You have likely spent the past nine months studying, listening, and absorbing all the advice and wisdom you can. You've done everything within your power to make your partner comfortable, and you are both on the same page about the delivery. While there are some symptoms that will continue in the ninth month, your main focus will be the preparation for labor and your strategy for the delivery day. You'll also want to decide on a name if you haven't yet; you and your partner have likely had this conversation, and you may have already chosen one well before the due date.

Labor can happen when you least expect it. When Leah went into labor with our first child she was cooking dinner for her mom on mother's day. She had been struggling with Braxton Hicks Contractions, and felt that familiar tight feeling. She kept making dinner, thinking that it was just another false alarm. Then, just as the oven timer was about to go off, her water broke. Leah called me, but I was parking at the truck yard and missed her call. I still have that voicemail saved on my phone, where she casually stated, "Hey Sweetie, soooo the baby's coming. Might want to pick up the phone, bye Nigel." I did return the call minutes later, and we got her to the hospital with plenty of time to spare. Her mom did have to eat hospital food for her mother's day meal, but she couldn't have been happier!

Luckily, we had copies of our birth plan in the car and everything ready to go. The key to the delivery day is preparation. Make sure if you have other children, there is a place for them to go, and any pets you have are looked after. You'll also want to pack ahead of time. First, let's look at how the baby will develop in the last month.

WHAT IS HAPPENING TO THE BABY DURING THE NINTH MONTH?

While the focus of the ninth month tends to be on the delivery day, your baby is still developing right up until they are ready to be born. Your baby's lungs will continue to form until birth, and will be ready to take in that first breath once delivered. Your child will also have packed on another 1 or 2 pounds since the last month, and grown between 1 and 2.5 inches in length.

The baby will also begin to move into a head-down position known as vertex presentation: this is so the child will be born head-first and be able to start breathing in air. If the baby doesn't make this movement, they'll be in what's known as a breech position, which may lead to complications. There are tests that can detect whether your baby is in the right position and a healthcare professional can attempt to position the baby manually. Your doctor may also recommend a cesarean birth to prevent any complications from occurring.

In preparing for the big day, you'll want to make sure you prepack every item your partner and newborn will need. Here is a checklist you can follow to make sure nothing is forgotten.

HOSPITAL PACKING CHECKLIST

You'll want to start packing all necessary bags before the due date, so they are ready to go the moment your partner goes into labor. Some items you won't be able to pack early, which is understandable; have a list posted in a convenient area and an empty bag at the ready, so you can pack these items quickly. There are several types of bags you'll need to pack, one for your newborn and several for your spouse.

What To Pack For Your Newborn

While the baby won't require too much at first, there are some items that will be absolutely necessary to bring to the hospital. These are usually related to the baby's safety, health, and nutrition.

- Swaddles and Blankets: While the hospital will provide swaddles and blankets, they will not be made of the softest material. Packing your own blankets can help protect your newborn from the cold while making sure their skin isn't irritated by rough material. Bringing your own blankets also eliminates the need to move your newborn from the hospital-provided material to your own.

- Car Seat: Not only is a car seat the best way to protect your newborn on the ride home, it's also required in many places to leave the hospital at all. The nurses that help take your partner out to your car will only allow you to leave if they see a car seat installed inside of your vehicle. Make sure the car seat you purchase has ample padding and faces the rear section of your car.

- Clothes: Make sure to pack some clothes for the baby to wear once you leave the hospital. Check the weather reports for the days near the delivery and pack accordingly; if it's cold, a jacket, hat, and warm socks will be essential. You'll also want to pack burp cloths for when your baby begins to spit up. Burp cloths can help reduce the number of times you have to change the baby's clothes, as they will probably be spitting up a lot.

- Bottles and Formula: The hospital will usually provide bottles and formula, but they may not match up with the diet plan you have for your child. Make sure to ask the hospital ahead of time, and plan on bringing your own.
- Diapers: Again, the hospital may provide a few diapers, but it's always good to bring extra. The hospital diapers may also be a bit lower quality, and packing soft and absorbent diapers on your own is the best course of action. You'll also want to pack some lotion and diaper rash cream to soothe your baby's delicate skin.

What To Pack For Your Partner

Your newborn will definitely be a priority, but making sure your spouse has everything they need is equally as important. There are many items you'll need to pack for your partner, including:

- Paperwork: Filling out paperwork ahead of time can help remove a lot of the anxiety associated with birth. Documentations like admittance forms or insurance information are best handled before the due date, so you can have one less thing to worry about when you arrive at the hospital.

- Birth Plan: We talked about having a birth plan in chapter 7, but there's one step I didn't mention: make sure to bring it with you! Having a copy, or even two, of your plan in your bags can help in those moments where you may be panicking. Make sure to give a copy to the head of your care team and any doctors or nurses working with your partner. That way, everyone will be on the same page.

- Identification: Make sure to bring identification for both you and your partner. This includes ID like driver's licenses, state ID cards, military ID, or your passport.

- Insurance: The hospital will require you to have all insurance information when you arrive, though it's usually best to provide them with insurance details before your delivery date.

- Comfortable Clothes: Comfortable clothes include everything your partner will need during labor and delivery: that means maternity clothes to wear home, a nursing gown to wear during breastfeeding, and a nursing bra to wear under their hospital gown.

- Comfort Item: Your partner will likely be stressed, so if they have any sort of comfort item make sure to pack it. This can be a childhood blanket or stuffed animal, a silly picture that makes them laugh, or a scent that makes them comfortable. Talk with your partner ahead of time about what would put them at ease, and make sure to pack it before leaving for the hospital.
- Cell phone and charger: You'll want to take pictures and videos of your newborn to send to friends and family, and you can't do that with a dead phone. Make sure to grab both you and your partner's cell phones and their requisite chargers. You'll also want your phone to keep in contact with family during labor and delivery.
- Glasses or contacts: Depending on whether your partner has eye-impairments, glasses or contacts may be necessary to bring to the hospital. If they do have contacts, make sure to also pack contact lens solution.
- Lip balm: Hospitals can be a very dry environment, and a little lip balm can help prevent your partner from suffering from cracked and chapped lips.
- Water and snacks: Staying hydrated and staving away hunger are important parts of keeping

your partner happy and stress-free. Pack a couple of water bottles and some healthy snacks, as food may not be the hospital's priority when you first arrive.

- Medications: Any medications that your partner is prescribed, whether pregnancy-related or not, should be packed in your hospital bags. Make sure to inform your care team about what medications your partner is on, so they can see if they interact with anything she'll be given in the hospital.

- Sleep mask and ear plugs: You and your partner will likely spend at least one night in the hospital. Sleeping in these facilities can be difficult, as there is usually some type of light or noise happening at all hours. A sleep mask and ear plugs can make this uncomfortable experience a bit easier.

- Toiletries: You should pack the toiletries you would usually take on a trip, like toothpaste, toothbrush, soap, deodorant, shampoo, and a hairbrush. Consider taking a towel and flip flops in case you or your partner need a shower.

GETTING TO THE HOSPITAL

Once you get to the hospital, it's just a matter of following your birth plan and listening to the advice of your care team. There really isn't much to do during labor but stay with your partner, comfort them, and follow any instructions given by your doctor. Make sure not to get in the way, and allow the doctors to give your wife the best care possible.

Listen closely to your spouse and provide them with anything they ask for (in my experience, this is mainly ice chips and to squeeze your hand until it hurts).

You can help your partner by:

- Massaging your partner's temples
- Give her cold compressed to cool her down
- Help her get to the bathroom
- Provide her with any items she needs from the packed bags
- Assist her in moving when she gets uncomfortable
- Listen! If she asks you to move away, you *have* to. Do whatever you can to provide her with maximum comfort
- Apply heat to her lower back if she's in pain
- Gently remind her to breathe

- After the birth, manage the amount of guests in the room while your partner and the baby are resting. Too many people can be overstimulating after an experience as intense as delivery, it's time for mom and baby to rest

Labor can last anywhere from several hours to 2 days, so prepare yourself mentally for the intensity of this event. The best part is, it all culminates in you seeing your child for the first time, which is truly a life-changing moment. Don't be worried if your initial reaction isn't what you hoped: When I first looked at Alan, he didn't look real. Babies look a bit strange when they are first born, and Alan was purple, red, and covered in afterbirth.

But as they washed him and handed him to Leah in a little blanket, all I could think was "This little guy is going to be my everything. I can't wait to get to know him." I said his name, and he immediately looked at me like he recognized me. Maybe all those months of whispering to my wife's belly had gotten in his ears, or maybe I was just delirious from lack of sleep, but I felt an instant connection. And my prediction was right; He really is my everything, and over the last 10 years I've gotten to know him very well.

FROM WATERMELON, TO IN YOUR ARMS (THIS LITTLE CHILD OF OURS)

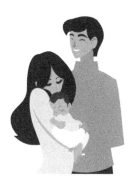

"Daddy loves you."

-Craig Bartlett, as the voice of Miles Shortman on Hey Arnold!

VOCABULARY FOR NEWBORN CARE:

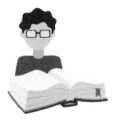

in·fant	cra·dle
/ˈinfənt/	/ˈkrādl/
noun	*noun*
A very young child or baby.	1. An infant's bed or crib, typically one mounted on rockers.
	verb
	2. Hold gently and protectively.

sha·ken ba·by syn·drome	bonding
/SHāken ˈbābē ˈsinˌdrōm/	/ˈbändiNG/
noun	*verb*
A condition characterized by cranial injury, retinal hemorrhage, etc. observed in infants who have been violently shaken or jolted.	The establishment of a relationship or link with someone based on shared feelings, interests, or experiences.

um·bil·i·cal cord	sud·den in·fant death syn·drome
/ˌəmˈbilək(ə)l ˌkôrd/	
noun	/ˈsədn ˈinfənt deTH ˈsinˌdrōm/
A flexible cordlike structure containing blood vessels and attaching a human or other mammalian fetus to the placenta during gestation.	noun
	The death of a seemingly healthy baby in its sleep, due to an apparent spontaneous cessation of breathing.

chafe	breast milk
/CHāf/	/ˈbrest ˌmilk/
verb	noun
(Of something restrictive or too tight) make (a part of the body) sore by rubbing against it.	Milk produced by a woman's breasts after childbirth as food for her child.

WELCOMING YOUR NEWBORN

The pregnancy is officially over, and you are holding your new son or daughter in your arms. So what's next? While taking care of a child is more than I can fit in a chapter, I do want to talk a bit about what to do with your newborn in the first few weeks.

You've left the hospital, and are ready to bring your newborn home to start your brand new life as a family man. First off, congratulations to both you and your partner! It took a lot to get here, and there is certainly plenty of work ahead, but you have both successfully navigated the difficult and rewarding process of pregnancy.

What Will the Baby Look Like?

The first thing you may notice about your child is that they look a bit...weird. Newborns aren't something we see a lot in the media, which is good; newborn babies don't need to be in commercials and on TV, they have important baby things to do. The problem with this lack of representation is that we often have a certain idea of how our child will look right after they're born: wide eyed, excited, lots of movement. The reality is, besides a near infinite ability to cry, newborns won't move too much for the first few days.

Their head may also be a bit pointy from their passage through the birth canal and will be quite a bit bigger than their body. The baby's skin can be very red for the first couple of days, and may be coated in vernix caseosa, a white skin-protectant created in the womb to protect a fetus from amniotic fluid. The baby's skin will likely be incredibly wrinkly, and their limbs may seem awkwardly positioned and bent. All of these are brief after-effects from their gestation, and will fade in the coming weeks.

BREASTFEEDING AND LATCHING

For the first 24 hours, you'll want to wake your baby every 2 to three hours to feed them. Your partner may have difficulty producing breast milk for the first couple of days, and will instead produce colostrum. Colostrum is a breast-milk precursor, and is usually a thin and watery substance. If the colostrum comes out thick and yellowish, there is no reason to worry; this is a less common but still natural form of pre breast-milk. There is a possibility that the baby will have a difficult time latching, which is the act of getting suction onto the breast.

If your baby is not latching properly there are several steps you can take, including:

- The Tickle Method: One way to help your baby latch onto the nipple is to tickle the baby's lips with the nipple itself. Baby's have a natural instinct to react to the physical connection, and will hopefully open their mouth to feed.
- Adjust The Baby's Head Position: Sometimes the issue is that the baby isn't angled properly to latch. Try aiming the nipple just above the baby's upper lip, and make sure the baby's head is angled up and away from their chest.

- Fish Lips: Another way to get a baby to latch is to make sure their lips are facing outward like a fish. You want to aim the baby away from the base of the nipple, and get them to latch onto the nipple chin first. The baby's tongue should extend as the breast fills up their mouth; hopefully, they'll then latch and start feeding.
- Move to a Calm Environment: Make sure your partner has a room they feel comfortable in, one that is quiet with gentle lighting. You can even help set a calming mood with gentle music and scented candles, making sure to take away anything that may disturb the baby.
- Let the Baby Go At Their Own Pace: It's natural to want to help guide our baby to latch, but babies are programmed to instinctually breastfeed. Have your partner try offering her breast to the baby but not put their nipple into the baby's mouth. Eventually, your newborn should grow curious and latch on their own accord.

You'll know a baby is properly latched onto the breast if your partner is comfortable and doesn't feel any excessive biting. The baby should be at rest with their chest and stomach pressed gently against the body. Their chin will be touching the breast, and their mouth will be around the entire breast and not just the nipple. You'll know that the baby has begun feeding when you see or hear them swallowing; a slight movement in the ears can also be a sign that the baby is successfully feeding.

CHANGING DIAPERS

Though it's no one's favorite task, changing diapers will be a major part of your life for the foreseeable future. It can be a bit tough at first, and a little gross, but eventually you'll be able to change their diaper with your eyes closed. You'll build this skill quickly as well, because babies can go through upwards of 10 diapers in a single day.

To start, you'll want to get everything you'll need for a diaper change, including:

- Diapers (of course)
- Baby wipes
- Diaper cream
- Garbage bag
- Change of clothes (for the baby, but if things go really bad, for you as well)
- A changing table or pad

Step 1: Prepare your supplies and environment

Make sure to have everything you need close by and set up for easy use. Make sure the changing table or pad is clean, and there is nothing within the baby's reach that they can grab during the changing. Wash your hands before beginning so they are clean when you touch your newborn.

Step 2: Remove the dirty diaper

Once your baby has been placed on their back on the changing table, loosen the tabs on either side of their diaper. Once the tabs are unfastened, grasp your newborn's ankles and bottom and gently lift them out of the soiled diaper. If the diaper is especially dirty you can use the upper half to gently push the stool towards the lower half. Then, slide the diaper away and place it out of reach of your baby.

Step 3: Clean and sanitize

Using the baby wipes, clean the entire area covered by the diaper. If you have a daughter make sure to wipe their vulva from front to back. If done incorrectly, your baby could develop an infection, so make sure to clean the area fully. Once you are done, dispose of the baby wipes in the same area as the dirty diaper.

Step 4: Place the clean diaper

Once the entire area is cleaned and spotless, gently lift your baby and slide a clean diaper under their bottom. The tabs on the diaper should be under the child, and most diapers have markings to indicate which side faces front. Don't close the diaper quite yet though! You want to apply the diaper cream to help prevent any rashes from developing. You shouldn't use any baby powder, as this can get inhaled by the baby and cause lung irritation.

Once the cream is applied, close the diaper. Pull the front of the diaper between your newborn's legs and over their stomach, pulling the tabs open and around to the front. Make sure not to put the diaper on too tightly, as this can cause the baby discomfort. If your baby still has their umbilical stump (which is likely in the first couple of days) make sure to fold the diaper down to avoid disturbing the stump.

Step 5: Finish and clean the area

Roll the dirty diaper and used baby wipes up and close the tabs, placing the diaper in your garbage bag and sealing it tight. Disinfect any changing surface; this will not only prevent contamination but will also help prevent any lingering smell that can be left behind.

Wash both you and your baby's hands, and then you are done!

Don't be alarmed by the appearance of the baby's poop in the first week or two. A newborn's stool looks very different from ours, and can appear a greenish-black color, yellow, or the usual brown. You may also see a rusty red substance known as urate crystals. These are a result of the high protein in breast milk, which can cause a rise in acidic urine. This acidity forms crystals, which are then transferred into the diaper. While these crystals can be normal, seeing them too often can be a cause for concern. An abundance of urate crystals indicates that a baby is experiencing dehydration, and it may be best to call your pediatrician.

Look for the signs of dehydration, which include:

- Dry skin
- A reduced amount of wet diapers in 24 hour period
- Dark brown or unusually yellow urine
- Crying, but with no tears being produced by the tear ducts

BONDING WITH THE BABY

While the process of biological bonding is mainly for the mother and baby, you can help by educating yourself about the proper bonding procedures. Don't confuse this for regular bonding, which is still an important part about being a parent. The bond formed between a mother and child has direct benefits to both your partner and your infant. Bonding can lower the stress levels of the mother and child and can start to grow a trusting, lifelong attachment between parent and child.

There are ways your partner can bond with the baby, including:

- *Playing:* While you have to be very careful with an infant, there are ways you can keep them engaged and get those synapses firing. Placing them in an interesting environment, giving them a rattle or other safe toy, or reading them stories with vibrant pictures are all great ways to bond with your infant.
- *Bottle-feeding:* Bottle feeding is an excellent time for the baby to get used to your partner's scent and touch. There is a common misconception that bottle-feeding can negatively affect bonding, but this isn't true: The act of feeding

and the hormones within the breast milk are the main factors that facilitate bonding.

- *Breastfeeding:* Breastfeeding has the advantage of giving the child and mother skin-skin contact, and can be a more affectionate process than bottle-feeding. The drawback would be that breastfeeding can be hard on your partner's nipples, and may cause them pain after multiple feedings.

- *Holding:* Touch is the most important sense associated with bonding, and a combination of holding and eye-contact can help improve communication. Your baby will begin to imitate your facial expressions, and follow your movements with their eyes. This all helps facilitate their social development later in life.

- *Vocalizing:* Babies are naturally attuned to the human voice, and will delight in listening to you speak, sing, or read aloud. You and your partner should both talk with your baby early and often; this will help them grow accustomed to the sound of your voice and automatically seek it out.

TAKE A MOMENT TO ASSESS

Once you've taken all the steps to get the baby situated, take a second to take stock of you and your partner's mental health. Labor and delivery is an incredibly stressful experience, and a crying newborn may only exacerbate any tension you both already feel. Ask your partner if they need anything, and try to take care of any physical ailments they are feeling. Make sure you are both hydrated, and if possible take turns taking a short nap to fight the effects of sleep deprivation. It can be difficult with all the adrenaline and energy you'll feel seeing your child, but exhaustion can lead to mistakes.

It's also good to look for the signs of postpartum depression. It's natural to feel a bit of sadness after a birth, as your partner's hormones will still be fluctuating widely and the process of labor is very intense on the body. This sadness can persist for a few weeks, but will usually fade. If it doesn't it could signal they are suffering from postpartum depression. Postpartum depression is a condition many mothers face shortly after birth, and can result in sudden crying, overwhelming anxiety, mood swings, and insomnia. If these symptoms occur they usually start between two and four days after the baby is born, and can last for many months. If you find that your partner is feeling depressed for more than a few weeks post-delivery, you

184 | NIGEL BOYD

should consult a psychologist to see if they need any extra help.

SUDDEN INFANT DEATH SYNDROME AND PREVENTION TIPS

While it's not a subject most people don't want to think about, sudden infant death syndrome or SIDs is a reality all parents should work to prevent. The good news is the rate of SIDS has been steadily falling since the mid 1990's, and usually only occurs in newborns with brain defects, low birth weight, or a respiratory infection. That being said, it's still essential to take all the steps possible for your own peace of mind.

While there is no 100% guaranteed way to prevent SIDs, here are several tips you can use to help your baby sleep more safely.

Tip #1: Spacious Crib

Try to get a decent sized crib for your child, one that has a firm mattress. This will keep the baby from sinking down into soft material, which can interfere with their breathing. While it can be hard to keep a baby away from their stuffed animals, large fluffy toys should be kept out of the crib. These too can obstruct your child's breathing if they end up in an unusual sleeping position.

Tip #2: Back to Sleep

Speaking of sleep, you may have heard the term "back to sleep" before. The initial position you put your baby in during sleep is important, and it can be easy to think the baby can simply sleep the same way we do: On our stomach, side, or back. But for infants, the absolute best way to ensure a safe sleep is to put them on their back. If you have others take care of the child, whether that be a loved one or a nanny, make sure to inform anyone who puts the baby to sleep to put the child on their back.

Tip #3: Watch the Temperature

It's natural to want to make sure your baby is sleeping in a warm enough environment, but it's important to never put any sort of headwear on your infant while they are sleeping. While these articles of clothing can cover ears and stop heat from escaping through the baby's head, it can also slip down and obstruct their breathing. You also don't want your baby to get over-heated, so it's best not to have too many layers over them as they sleep.

Tip #4: Keep a Close Watch

If it's at all possible, keep your child's crib inside of your room. This allows you to keep a better eye on your infant while they are sleeping. Try to keep this up for at least six months, and if you must have your child in a different room, make sure to use a baby monitor. If you do keep your child in your room, make sure they stay in their crib. While it may be tempting to let your baby sleep with you and your partner, this can be incredibly dangerous. The wide open and unsecured space surrounding an adult bed can give a baby any number of ways to become trapped; it's much safer for them to sleep in their crib.

NEVER BE AFRAID TO ASK FOR HELP

No matter how long I've been a father, I never fail to run into issues that require outside help. Not every answer is in a book, and you'll often want to seek the wisdom of those who have ample experience with parenting. I'll wrap up this chapter with a little story about my father, and how frustration is part of the parenting process.

My dad told me a story about a time when I was a child, and I had become fascinated with bringing bugs in the house to make them tiny makeshift houses. I thought they were my friends, and to be fair, it's never been proven they weren't. As good as my youthful intentions were in trying to build affordable housing for insects, this was obviously a hobby my parents would prefer I leave outdoors. They tolerated it for a short time, until the bugs started to take over.

My mother was woken up one night by a small group of grasshoppers that had escaped my room and snuck onto her pillow. A beetle surprised my Dad by crawling into his dinner, revealing itself as he went in for that first bite. Long story short, my parents weren't happy. They tried to reason with me and explain why I couldn't bring insects into the house, but they were my friends-so I persisted in my bug-helping habit. This continued until one day my father found a small colony of worms nestled in the bathroom and he lost his temper. He yelled, I cried, and he apologized shortly after. The part of the story I didn't know until later was what was going on at the time, and what my father did after his outburst.

It turns out during my strange insect housing phase, my parents were struggling with some financial issues. My dad wanted to have the patience to explain to me why my behavior was destructible, but he wasn't sure how to deal with my stubbornness, and he was already exhausted from working overtime. So he met his dad, my grandpa, at a local park for some fatherly advice. While the problem seemed silly, the piece of advice he gave seemed to work for many of the problems that face parents. Anytime I get frustrated with one of my kids or make a mistake, I remember his words and try to give myself a bit of a break.

"Be patient," my grandpa said, "So many people aren't, and they always suffer for it. You're a young man, this is all so new to you. Balancing a job, wife, kids, learning how to do all of that is a learning curve. It won't happen in a month or even a year, but eventually you'll be sitting where I am, giving your kid advice. I promise that, eventually, you'll have this figured out. All it takes is time."

FREE GIFT!

As a thank you for purchasing my book, here is a gift.
Scan the QR code and enjoy!'

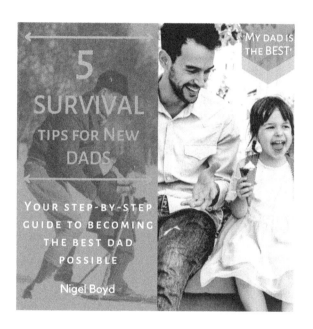

AFTERWORD

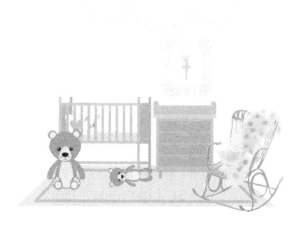

Making it through a pregnancy is a major achievement for both you and your partner, and it's important to take the time to acknowledge the huge accomplishment you've both completed. The first couple of months after the baby is born will be hectic, and you may not be ready to let someone else watch them quite yet. But if possible, take a weekend to get away with your spouse and reflect on the last year. Ask yourselves some questions about each trimester of the pregnancy, what your expectations were, what were some of the bigger hurdles, what you would do differently, and what were your favorite moments. Let's take a look at some introspective questions as you welcome your child into your home.

QUESTIONS TO ASK AFTER THE PREGNANCY

- *What were your expectations for the pregnancy?*

If you've been keeping a journal, you'll be able to go back and look at your thoughts from those first couple of months. You'll see that many of the major fears you were having may have been a bit overblown, while other issues you didn't see coming popped up. As time went on, you can see how those more existential worries (Will my child be a good person, will I be able to provide, am I ready to be a dad) fade away as you focus on the here-and-now. Many couples find that by focusing on creating a healthy pregnancy for the baby, and a stress-free environment for the mother, those longer-term concerns get put in perspective.

Many couples also underestimate the sheer amount of small tasks that constitute proper baby preparation. From finding baby clothes to making your home safe to deciding on whether or not to be a stay at home parent, there are hundreds of tiny things you'll need to do you probably didn't even consider. Some parts of pregnancy that you thought would be far more important, like naming the baby, fall to the way-side as you try to find the right doctors, construct a clear birth plan, and deal with the numerous physical symptoms. After your first pregnancy, you'll find that your expectations will be far different for any future children.

- *What were some of the biggest hurdles?*

Both you and your partner will have different answers for this question, and it's always interesting to consider both sides of the pregnancy experience when looking at the biggest hurdles. For your wife, the physical symptoms were likely one of the more difficult parts of the pregnancy. The strain a pregnancy puts on a woman's body is tremendous, with fatigue and nausea making some days very uncomfortable. For you, the biggest problems were probably psychological. Worrying about your partner, whether everything would be ready for the baby, how the labor and delivery would go. By looking at what your big struggles were in your first pregnancy, you can often prepare yourself better in the future. I'll give you an example.

One symptom both me and Leah agreed on being incredibly stressful were Braxton Hicks contractions. With our first child, these false alarms would always send both of us into fits of anxiety. I noticed on our second go around though, we both took them in stride. As we grew more accustomed to the differences between Braxton Hicks and real contractions, it was easy to recognize the signs. Take the time to look at your own biggest issues, and see what you each struggled with and what overlapped. Talking about these concerns can help bring you both onto the same page for future pregnancies.

- *What would you do differently?*

It's difficult for everyone to self-assess and determine what they could have done better during a pregnancy. Maybe you and your partner let the stress get to you and fought on occasion. Maybe you weren't able to eliminate some of your habits, and weren't able to show solidarity to your partner as they stopped theirs. It's possible there were some activities, like consistent exercise, that you both just were not able to keep up on. Establishing a list of things you would have liked to do better can help you determine how to be better in the future. Making mistakes is part of being human, and a huge part of being a parent. Learning to look inward and find out how you can do better is a great skill to learn, and can help you make better parenting decisions in the future.

- *What were your favorite moments?*

While pregnancy can be stressful, it is also a uniquely exciting part of the human experience. Sure, there will be times when you are so tired you can't focus, you're holding back your wife's hair as she vomits, or you've become frustrated with endless doctors appointments and confusing medical terminology. It's important to find the parts of the pregnancy you liked, and help reinforce those memories by discussing them with your partner.

For our first pregnancy, Leah and I both agreed that many aspects were incredible. The baby shower was a blast, and those little moments like walking in the mornings and finding ways to satisfy Leah's strange and often humorous pregnancy cravings were highlights, but the babymoon was an especially wonderful and special time for both of us. I talked about it briefly in chapter 6, but to briefly recap we took some time to ourselves to visit Banff National Park in Canada. The snow capped mountains sitting calmly in the background as we laughed and ate cheese, huddled around a fireplace, is one of our most cherished memories of all time! Talk with your partner about what parts of the pregnancy you both loved, and try to solidify one of these memories together. This could be done by preserving any pictures or videos you took during the trip, maybe in a scrapbook or short edited home movie. Whatever way you choose, make sure to hold on to those special moments for the rest of your life.

WHAT I WANT YOU TO TAKE AWAY

My hope with this book was to give you as much of the knowledge I've accrued over the years as possible. Pregnancy can be such an arduous journey, and having even a bit more of an idea what lies ahead can make the experience so much easier. Of course, you'll have your own way of doing things, and that's more than okay. I certainly didn't follow the advice of every book I read to a T, and how you help your partner and child is ultimately up to you. Despite all the experts and books on the subject, there is no single correct way to be a parent. A lot of times you'll need to trust your gut, and do what you think is right for your loved ones. Make your family's story one of a kind.

If you enjoyed this book, it would mean the world to me if you would leave a review on Amazon. I think that the information stored here can really help out first time dads, and I'm certain the time I spent compiling everything was well worth it. I continue to do research to this day, and I plan to continue this series in the hope I can help as many dads as possible.

It can be strange to look back all those months ago and think about that first moment. It may be a bit hard to picture now, but try to remember where you were. Driving in your car, sitting at work, or even looking into the eyes of your partner, seconds before you would hear the sentence that would change your life forever. You can think about it now, as you hold your newborn, how far you've come from those six little words; You're going to be a dad. And now that you made it through the nine months of trials and tribulations, you'll be presented with a new sentence. A bit shorter, but no less powerful.

You are a dad.

A Note To My Readers: Thank you for reading 'I'm Gonna Be A First-Time Dad'! Please leave a review, I'd greatly appreciate the feedback so that I can continue to help awesome future dad's like *yourself*.

RESOURCES

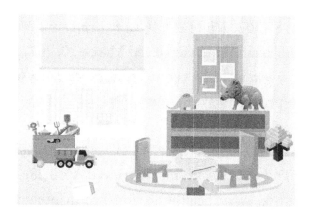

20 things you need to know about your newborn. (n.d.). News 24. Retrieved April 17, 2022, from https://www.news24.com/parent/baby/babycare/newborn/20-things-you-need-to-know-about-your-newborn-20160421

AboutKidsHealth. (n.d.-a). About Kids Health. Retrieved April 27, 2022, from https://www.aboutkidshealth.ca/ Article?contentid=319&language=English

AboutKidsHealth. (n.d.-b). About Kids Health. Retrieved March 28, 2022, from https://www.aboutkidshealth. ca/Article?contentid=320&language=English

AboutKidsHealth. (n.d.-c). About Kids Health. Retrieved April 17, 2022, from https://www.aboutkidshealth.ca/ Article?contentid=327&language=English

Bradley, S. (2020a, July 29). *What to Expect at 6 Months Pregnant*. Health Line. Retrieved March 20, 2022, from https://www.healthline.com/health/pregnancy/6-months-pregnant#symptoms

Bradley, S. (2020b, October 16). *What to Expect at 5 Months Pregnant*. Healthline. Retrieved April 28, 2022, from https://www.healthline.com/health/pregnancy/ 5-months-pregnant#see-a-doctor

Brien, A., MD. (2021, February 5). *5 common questions about Braxton Hicks contractions*. Mayo Clinic Health System. Retrieved March 22, 2022, from https://www. mayoclinichealthsystem.org/hometown-health/speak ing-of-health/5-common-questions-about-braxton-

hicks-contractions#:%7E:text=Braxton%20Hicks%
20contractions%20are%20mild

Crider, C. (2021, May 25). *What to Expect at 8 Months Pregnant.* Health Line. Retrieved April 17, 2022, from https://www.healthline.com/health/pregnancy/8-months-pregnant#fetal-development

familyeducation.com. (2021a, December 14). *Month Two of Your Pregnancy.* Family Education. Retrieved April 27, 2022, from https://www.familyeducation.com/preg nancy/first-trimester/month-two-your-pregnancy

familyeducation.com. (2021b, December 15). *You are 9 Weeks Exactly Pregnant.* Family Education. Retrieved March 20, 2022, from https://www.familyeducation. com/pregnancy/week-9-pregnancy/you-are-9-weeks-exactly-pregnant

The First Day of Life (for Parents) - Nemours KidsHealth. (n.d.). Kids Health. Retrieved April 17, 2022, from https://kidshealth.org/en/parents/first-day.html

A Guide for First-Time Parents (for Parents) - Nemours KidsHealth. (n.d.). Kids Health. Retrieved April 17, 2022, from https://kidshealth.org/en/parents/guide-parents.html

Herndon, M. J. S. (2019, March 8). *10 Home Remedies for Swollen Feet*. Healthline. Retrieved March 22, 2022, from https://www.healthline.com/health/home-reme dies-for-swollen-feet

How music affects your baby's brain: Mini Parenting Master Class. (n.d.). UNICEF Parenting. Retrieved April 5, 2022, from https://www.unicef.org/parenting/child-development/how-music-affects-your-babys-brain-class#:%7E:text=What%20music%20should%20a%20pregnant

How to Change a Diaper. (2022, February 9). Verywell Family. Retrieved March 28, 2022, from https://www.verywellfamily.com/how-to-change-a-diaper-289239

Hunterdon Healthcare. (2019a, November 14). *Services for Pregnancy Eighth Month*. Retrieved March 28, 2022, from https://www.hunterdonhealthcare.org/service/maternity/pregnancy-month-by-month/pregnancy-eighth-month/

Hunterdon Healthcare. (2019b, November 14). *Services for Pregnancy Fifth Month*. Retrieved April 28, 2022, from https://www.hunterdonhealthcare.org/service/maternity/pregnancy-month-by-month/pregnancy-fifth-month/

Kobola, F. (2017a, March 10). *10 Thoughts a Guy Has When He Finds Out He's Going to be a Dad.* Cosmopolitan. Retrieved April 27, 2022, from https://www.cosmopolitan.com/sex-love/a9114672/thoughts-guys-have-about-fatherhood/

Kobola, F. (2017b, March 10). *10 Thoughts a Guy Has When He Finds Out He's Going to be a Dad.* Cosmopolitan. Retrieved April 27, 2022, from https://www.cosmopolitan.com/sex-love/a9114672/thoughts-guys-have-about-fatherhood/

Mullen, A. (2020, December 8). *The Essential Newborn Baby Hospital Bag Checklist.* Mustela USA. Retrieved April 17, 2022, from https://www.mustelausa.com/blogs/mustela-mag/the-essential-newborn-baby-hospital-bag-checklist

My wife is pregnant. What advice do you have for a new father? (n.d.). Quora. Retrieved April 27, 2022, from https://www.quora.com/My-wife-is-pregnant-What-advice-do-you-have-for-a-new-father

N. (2021, June 8). *Symptoms of the first month of pregnancy.* Natalben. Retrieved March 22, 2022, from https://www.natalben.com/en/pregnancy-months/1-month-pregnant

Novak, S. C. W. (2022, March 22). *What Is a Midwife and Should You Hire One for Your Pregnancy and Baby's Birth?* What to Expect. Retrieved March 22, 2022, from https://www.whattoexpect.com/pregnancy/labor-and-delivery/hiring-midwife/#:%7E:text=Midwives%20are%20a%20good%20choice

Orloff, N. C. (2014). *Pickles and ice cream! Food cravings in pregnancy: hypotheses, preliminary evidence, and directions for future research.* Frontiers. Retrieved April 5, 2022, from https://www.frontiersin.org/articles/10.3389/fpsyg.2014.01076/full

Partner Support During Pregnancy | CS Mott Children's Hospital | Michigan Medicine. (n.d.). CS Mott Children's Hospital. Retrieved March 28, 2022, from https://www.mottchildren.org/health-library/abp7352

Pregnancy Calendar - Week by Week Stages | Pampers. (n.d.). Web-Pampers-US-EN. Retrieved March 22, 2022, from https://www.pampers.com/en-us/pregnancy/pregnancy-calendar

Slide show: Pregnancy stretches. (2020, November 24). Mayo Clinic. Retrieved March 28, 2022, from https://www.mayoclinic.org/healthy-lifestyle/pregnancy-

week-by-week/multimedia/pregnancy/sls-20076930?
s=6

Smoking, Pregnancy, and Babies. (n.d.). Centers for
Disease Control and Prevention. Retrieved April 27,
2022, from https://www.cdc.gov/tobacco/campaign/
tips/diseases/pregnancy.html#:%7E:text=Smoking%
20raises%20your%20baby

Staff, R. (2012, February 16). *One in 10 U.S. kids have
alcoholic parent: study.* Reuters. Retrieved April 27, 2022,
from https://www.reuters.com/article/us-usa-drink
ing-study/one-in-10-u-s-kids-have-alcoholic-parent-
study-idUSTRE81F0CB20120216

Stress and pregnancy. (n.d.). Stress and Pregnancy.
Retrieved November 7, 2021, from https://www.
marchofdimes.org/complications/stress-and-pregnancy.
aspx#:%7E:text=High%20levels%20of%20stress%20that

Tobacco Statistics & Facts. (n.d.). ASH > Action on
Smoking & Health. Retrieved April 27, 2022, from
https://ash.org/programs/tobacco-statistics-facts/?
gclid=CjwKCAiA55mPBhBOEiwANmzoQjNPM
PRvu8LF8vS3xggXTRlLu3gLisSqP_yuxb_AEmdZAw
PocJ6N-RoCrp8QAvD_BwE

UC Davis Health, Public Affairs and Marketing. (n.d.). *The Importance of Infant Bonding | UC Davis Medical Center.* UC Davis Medical Center. Retrieved March 28, 2022, from https://health.ucdavis.edu/medicalcenter/healthtips/20100114_infant-bonding.html#:%7E:text=Bonding%20is%20essential%20for%20normal

Understanding Miscarriage -- Prevention. (2002, November 1). WebMD. Retrieved March 22, 2022, from https://www.webmd.com/baby/understanding-miscarriage-prevention

Usa, M. (2020, July 31). *The Complete Pregnancy Checklist: A Month-By-Month Guide.* Mustela USA. Retrieved April 28, 2022, from https://www.mustelausa.com/blogs/mustela-mag/pregnancy-checklist

What Happens at 3 Months of Pregnancy? | 12 Weeks Pregnant. (n.d.). Planned Parenthood. Retrieved April 27, 2022, from https://www.plannedparenthood.org/learn/pregnancy/pregnancy-month-by-month/what-happens-third-month-pregnancy

What Is a Midwife? (n.d.). WebMD. Retrieved April 5, 2022, from https://www.webmd.com/baby/what-is-a-midwife-twins

What is a Miscarriage? | Causes of Miscarriage. (n.d.). Planned Parenthood. Retrieved April 5, 2022, from https://www.plannedparenthood.org/learn/preg nancy/miscarriage

Your Pregnancy: Month 7. (n.d.). The Tot. Retrieved April 17, 2022, from https://www.thetot.com/pregnancy-and-fertility/your-pregnancy-month-7-trimester/

Made in United States
Orlando, FL
20 December 2023

41292694R00125